D1179096

A Bicentennial Monograph On Hearing Impairment: Trends in the USA

Contents

Robert Frisina is the director of the National Technical Institute for the Deaf, Rochester, New York, a position held since the Institute's origination in 1967. He also serves as vice-president of the Rochester Institute of Technology and is currently chairman of the R.I.T. Board of Trustees' Commission on Institutional Advancement.

Throughout his career, Dr. Frisina's interest has been directed toward the education of deaf youth. His professional experience has included the roles of dean of the graduate school and director of the hearing and speech clinic at Gallaudet College, Washington, D.C., and UNESCO expert on the educational aspects of deafness in Hong Kong, as well as experience as an instructor of deaf children, audiologist, and clinician.

He is an active member of the A.G. Bell Association, functioning concurrently as a member of the Board of Directors and the Executive Committee, and chairman of the Planning Committee. Some of his other affiliations include membership in the Executive Committee, the Higher Education Committee, and chairman of the Committee to Redefine Deaf and Hard of Hearing for Educational Purposes of the Conference of Executives of American Schools for the Deaf; second vice-presidency of Highland Hospital, Rochester; and membership in the Medical Professional Advisory Committee of the Rochester Hearing and Speech Clinic.

Dr. Frisina has contributed to numerous textbooks and monographs on the subject of hearing impairment. His articles on speech, audiology, and the evolution of NTID have appeared in many professional journals, including the *American Annals of the Deaf, Exceptional Children,* and *The Volta Review.*

Introduction

It has been a tradition of the Alexander Graham Bell Association for the Deaf to bring to its members special issues of *The Volta Review* that can also be made available to professionals and policy-makers in related fields who look to the Association for information and recommendations. This Bicentennial Monograph, lucid in its somewhat comprehensive subject matter coverage and its extensive bibliography, should be of special interest to undergraduate and graduate students in speech pathology, audiology, special education, education of the hearing impaired, and to teachers in regular schools who are considering the inclusion of hearing impaired students in their classes.

In this Bicentennial year it seems appropriate to consider developments that have characterized the field of deafness in the past decade, and to project how these events, trends, and changes may affect the future for hearing impaired individuals into the 1980's.

It was once said, that "to renew ties with the past need not always be daydreaming. It may be tapping old sources of strength for new tasks." This monograph on two counts renews ties with the past, for it has been cast in the Bicentennial mold and it identifies with the legacy of Alexander Graham Bell on the 100th anniversary of his invention of the telephone. And both of these—the concept of an "America," and the inventiveness of the man—deeply imbedded in these chapters, are sources of strength for the special field in which we labor.

Turn-of-the-century immigrants from Europe and those who preceded them saw in America opportunity, growth, and the right to be one's self—a place where diversity, without conformity, was not only tolerated but welcomed. This monograph is consistent with this theme of America.

By calling upon many professions, it is pluralistic in its approach.

By considering a variety of practices, it respects diversity and avoids parochialism.

By its willingness to be self-critical, it presents an open view.

By its documentation, it is authoritative without being dogmatic.

By contrasting hopes from accomplishments, it recognizes a "state of the art" that is less than perfect.

Paraphrasing a famous "America-watcher" of more than 100 years ago (Alexis de Tocqueville) may manifest the spirit of the contributors to this monograph...They (contributors to this monograph) have all a lively faith in the perfectability of deaf children. They judge that the diffusion of knowledge must necessarily be advantageous, and the consequences of ignorance fatal; they all consider the education and growth of deaf people as a body in the state of improvement, the profession as a changing scene, in which no practices are, or ought to be, permanent; and they admit that what appears to them today to be good, may be superseded by something better tomorrow. *Robert Frisina*

1
Michael E. Glasscock, III, M.D., F.A.C.S.

Medical Intervention

Dr. Glassock is clinical assistant professor of surgery (otology and neurotology), Vanderbilt University, Nashville, Tennessee

Successful medical intervention for the patient with a hearing loss depends upon many factors. The first step is to establish a diagnosis. This can only be accomplished by means of a careful diagnostic evaluation. Once the nature and severity of the loss have been documented, the proper method of medical management can begin.

In determining the etiology of a hearing impairment, it is essential to obtain an accurate history. The onset as well as the character of the loss is important to establish. Was it sudden or progressive in nature? Are both ears involved, or is it a unilateral problem?

Familiar hearing impairment can usually be pinpointed by a positive family history. When one or both of the parents have similar problems the answer is obvious; however, many times these genetic difficulties skip generations and detecting them may present a real challenge.

In a young child, it is extremely important to know the mother's gestational history. Rubella contracted by the mother during pregnancy is the most common and widely known offender, but any viral disease can be implicated. Ototoxic drugs taken by the mother in the first trimester have received increasing attention in recent years.

Even the events that occur in an infant's first days or weeks of life can affect the auditory system. Again, drugs and febrile illnesses are the prime offenders.

Once the history has been established, audiometric studies are indicated to determine the nature and extent of the hearing impairment.

The physical examination aids the physician in his attempt to establish a diagnosis. Just looking at the ear and examining the eardrum can many times alert the physician to the underlying cause of the hearing loss. Congenital closure of the external ear canal or a perforation of the tympanic membrane would be obvious to the examiner. It is particularly important with children to establish whether the

2

patient fits into one of the known medical syndromes associated with hearing loss, such as Alport's and Usher's Syndromes (4). In establishing such a diagnosis, special examinations must be performed on the neurologic and visual systems. In addition, other organ systems such as the genitourinary tract should be investigated. This is accomplished by urinalysis and certain blood studies.

Congenital syphilis remains a prevalent medical problem and can produce a severe sensorineural impairment. This disease can be easily diagnosed now by a special blood test known as the F.T.A. (Fluorescent Treponemal Antibodies). Once established as the cause of the hearing loss, it is sometimes possible to reverse the impairment with special medications.

X-rays of the temporal bone (in which the middle and inner ears are housed) are of particular value in establishing the etiology of many otologic problems. A special x-ray machine, available in this country for about 10 years, is extremely valuable for evaluating the inner ear because of the fine detail that can be obtained. The name of this machine is the polytome, and most large city hospitals have one available.

There are several inner ear syndromes that can be diagnosed by x-ray. A complete absence of the inner ear is known as a Michael defect while dilatation of the cochlear turns would be a Mondini Syndrome. Otosclerosis can involve the whole inner ear and produce a sensorineural loss. This diagnosis can be established with the polytome, and the administration of sodium fluoride has been shown to prevent progression of the hearing impairment (5).

Management of the Patient with a Hearing Loss

The last 20 years have seen some dramatic changes in the field of otologic diagnosis and treatment. New surgical procedures for conductive hearing impairments have been developed.

Corrective surgery for hearing loss was first attempted in the 1930's by Dr. Julius Lempert. These procedures, called fenestrations, were for otosclerosis and enjoyed great success. In the early 1950's, Dr. Samuel Rosen of New York began to mobilize the stapes, and later Dr. John Shea of Memphis began to remove it altogether. The stapedectomy is now the standardized operation for otosclerosis, and the results are predictable and lasting.

Also in the early 1950's, Drs. Wullstein and Zollner of Germany began to perform an operation known as the tympanoplasty. This procedure is used to repair a perforated eardrum. It is now possible to control chronic infection and to repair the ossicular chain to improve hearing. The operating microscope and new micro-instrumentation have made modern, effective otologic surgery possible.

In children, most conductive hearing losses are amenable to surgery. The most common cause of a conductive loss is serous ototis media. This condition occurs when the eustachian tube fails to function and the middle ear fills with a fluid. The dampening effect on the tympanic membrane produces a hearing loss ranging from 20 dB to 50 dB, depending upon the consistency of the fluid. The underlying eustachian tube problem may be due to allergic problems or enlarged adenoids. In some cases, myringotomies with removal of the fluid and insertion of ventilating tubes will give immediate relief of the conductive loss. In others, allergic management or an adenoidectomy may be necessary to prevent eustachian tube malfunction.

Congenital deformities of the ear canal and ossicular chain are fairly common in children. If the problem is bilateral, some attempt at surgical correction is made. The ear canal can be opened and a skin graft applied. The ossicular chain can be reconstructed and the tympanic membrane grafted. A child with a congenital conductive loss that is unilateral is usually not a candidate for surgery, as most children with one normal ear do very well and compensate for the one malfunctioning ear. There are some risks with surgery, especially to the facial nerve in a congenitally deformed ear, so it is not usually recommended that a child with a unilateral loss undergo surgery until 15 to 18 years of age. At this time, an intelligent decision concerning the risks, complications, and possible benefits of surgery can be made by the individual.

One must not forget that the origin of many conductive hearing losses is an accumulation of ear wax. This occurs in children and adults alike and the wax should be removed by a physician, either by irrigations or by suction aspiration from the ear canal.

In young children with a conductive hearing loss, one should be watchful for foreign bodies lodged in the ear canal. These should be removed by an otologist or otolaryngologist under microscopic control with the patient under general anesthesia.

At the present time, some progress is being made in the field of electronics as applied to the inner ear.

Early detection and standard amplification of hearing loss in children have been very effective in recent years. On the horizon are implantable hearing aids that will possibly have great advantages over conventional amplification. These aids will be surgically implanted in the middle ear with direct coupling to the stapes. Some work is being done in this field at the present time and there are a few patients using these aids now (1).

Certainly, one of the most exciting advances in the last five years has been the cochlear implant. There are about 20 patients in the United States at this writing who have cochlear implants in place and functioning. These individuals for the most part are profoundly deaf. To date, these electrical devices must be considered as aids to lipreading. They do not reproduce clear speech, but the patient with a cochlear implant can "hear" certain sounds. While these implants are early in their developmental stage, it would appear that in the years to come they may hold promise for some individuals with profound sensorineural deafness (3).

What the Future Holds for the Medical Aspects of Hearing Loss

While great strides have been made in the last 20 years in the treatment of all types of hearing loss, the future must hold some great advances. Much basic research is being done in an attempt to determine the method by which one hears. There have been many theories set forth, but the precise mechanism is still not known. Investigative surgery for progressive sensorineural hearing loss is being performed in some European and American centers (2), and there is evidence that some types of progressive nerve deafness can be altered by surgical intervention. In the years to come, it may be possible to operate on the inner ear with the success we now enjoy in the middle ear. The future of surgical improvement should be considered bright.

The possible applications of modern electronics to hearing loss seem endless. Miniaturization of electrical circuits and the increase in knowledge of the physiology of the inner ear and central nervous system will make practical, electronic ears available in the future.

One of the most important immediate goals of the otologic community must be professional and lay education. It is imperative that the general medical physician and pediatrician be made aware of the problems of hearing loss, and especially of the need for early detection and intervention of hearing impairment in children. If the general medical community does not know what help is available for their patients, the fruits of modern otologic research are less likely to be passed on to the public.

More emphasis should be placed on educating the man-in-the-street, so that he may be informed about hearing impairment and what can be done about it. National organizations concerned with hearing impaired individuals should sponsor campaigns aimed at educating the lay public.

Summary

The 1950's and 1960's witnessed a tremendous upsurge of interest among otologists in the surgical management of conductive hearing loss. New microscopic instrumentation and operative techniques made possible great strides in this field. The last decade has seen a renewed interest in the problems of sensorineural impairment. New diagnostic tests and equipment make it possible to determine the type and etiology of many sensorineural losses that previously went undiagnosed. The next decade will undoubtedly be a productive one in the area of electronic aids to hearing. ⚹

2

Walter E. Nance, M.D., Ph.D.

Studies of Hereditary Deafness: Present, Past, and Future

Dr. Nance is professor of medicine, pediatrics, and human genetics and chairman of the Department of Human Genetics, Medical College of Virginia, Richmond.

It has been know for many years that genetic factors play an important role in the causation of deafness. The classic study by E. A. Fay (2), *Marriages Among the Deaf in America*, which was published in 1898, two years before the rediscovery of Gregory Mendel's work, clearly indicated the familial nature of many cases of deafness. However, it has been only within the past 20 years that accurate methods have been devised to define with precision the magnitude of the genetic component of deafness. One of the most important insights, gained from recent research, is that hereditary deafness is not a single disease but a large group of genetically distinct disorders that have one common symptom. The ear is one of the most intricate structures in the human body. It requires the precise interaction of the "instructions" contained in literally hundreds of genes to provide the information that the developing embryo needs to form a normal ear; and consequently, defects involving any one of many different gene pairs can all result in hearing loss.

Patterns of Inheritance

Recessive Inheritance. Sorting out some of the many different types of genetic hearing loss has been one of the major accomplishments of clinical research on the causes of deafness; and at the present time more than 50 different genetic syndromes are known in which hearing loss may occur. Several approaches have been used to characterize different forms of genetic deafness. One important criterion is the pattern of inheritance. We now know that in about 84% of all the genetic cases, deafness is transmitted as a recessive trait. This means that, in order to be affected, a child must inherit a double dose of the same abnormal gene—one from each of

6

the parents. Usually, the parents have normal hearing since they are carriers of only a single dose of the abnormal gene. In cases where two individuals with recessive deafness marry, they will have affected children only if both parents have the same kind of recessive deafness. Because there are so many different kinds of recessive deafness—caused by gene pairs located on different pairs of chromosomes—at least 70% of all matings of this type result in children with normal hearing who are carriers of single abnormal genes for deafness located at two different chromosomal regions. Being a carrier of a recessive gene for deafness should not be a matter of great concern unless one's spouse or prospective spouse is a carrier of the same abnormal gene. It is now known that everyone is a carrier of at least three to five abnormal recessive genes, and we can estimate that no fewer than one person in eight carries a recessive gene for deafness. The reason why recessive deafness is not more common is that, even if both parents carry a recessive gene for deafness, the chances are good, unless they are close relatives, that the recessive genes they carry will be members of different gene pairs at different chromosomal locations, and in this case the child cannot inherit a double dose of the same gene. Even if both parents are carriers of the same recessive gene, the chances are only one in four that each child will be affected. Human families are becoming so small that many parents who are at risk will be lucky two or three times in a row. If, by chance, they never have an affected child, they may never know the risk they ran. In other families, although the deafness is genetic, there may be only one affected child, and in many cases of this type, it may be difficult if not impossible to be sure whether the deafness has a genetic or an environmental cause.

Dominant inheritance. In about 14% of the genetic cases, deafness is transmitted as a dominant trait. In these forms of deafness, only one abnormal gene is required for expression of the trait, and since that gene must have come from either the father or the mother, we would ordinarily expect one of the parents to be affected if the gene is fully expressed. On the average, one-half of the children of a parent with dominant deafness will inherit the single abnormal gene.

Sex-linked inheritance. In about 2% of the cases, deafness is determined by a gene carried on the X chromosome and is transmitted as a "sex-linked trait" in much the same way that hemophilia, color blindness, or the commonest form of muscular dystrophy are inherited. With traits that show an X-linked pattern of inheritance, males are affected but females are usually normal, since males have only one X chromosome (along with a smaller Y chromosome), while females have two X chromosomes. Any abnormal gene carried on the single X chromosome of a male will be fully expressed, whereas a female will ordinarily require a double dose of the abnormal gene in order to express the trait fully. Typically, the family will contain multiple affected males who are all related to each other through female relatives who are carriers of the X-linked gene.

Associated Abnormalities

A second approach to recognizing different forms of genetic deafness is to search for distinctive associated abnormalities. For example, some types of hereditary deafness are associated with pigmentary abnormalities (18, 19), while others are associated with visual impairment (16), heart defects (4), thyroid abnormalities (3), kidney disease (10), or skeletal malformations (14), to mention a few. When present, these signs may permit the diagnosis of a specific hereditary deafness syndrome even when there is no other history of deafness in the family.

Considerable progress has also been made in defining certain forms of hereditary hearing loss by their audiologic characteristics. We know that some forms of deafness are associated with abnormalities in the organ of balance in the inner ear, while others are not. In some forms of genetic hearing loss, the high tones are preferentially affected (6) whereas in others low tone perception is lost (15). Finally, most forms of hereditary deafness lead to sensorineural loss. However, there is a small subgroup in which the hearing loss is conductive. This subgroup is particularly important to recognize because of the potential benefit affected individuals might receive from surgery or sound amplification.

Prevention and Treatment

Except for the syndromes that are associated with conductive loss, there are a few forms of hereditary deafness for which specific treatment is currently available. Refsum's syndrome is a rare, genetically determined neurologic disease, associated with hearing loss, in which a special low-phytanic-acid diet seems to be helpful (13). It is interesting that a genetically determined inner-ear abnormality in the mouse can be prevented by putting the pregnant mother on a special diet that is high in manganese. In several syndromes, treatment of associated abnormalities can be beneficial. For example, in the Jervell Lange-Neilsen syndrome (5), cardiac treatment can prevent the sometimes fatal fainting attacks; in Usher's syndrome (17), an early diagnosis of the retinitis pigmentosa can permit anticipatory educational planning. Specific forms of treatment for particular deafness syndromes will doubtless continue to be developed in the future. However, it seems unlikely that there will be a major "breakthrough" that will permit effective treatment for all forms of hereditary deafness. One form of sensorineural deafness that would seem to be a particularly attractive candidate for the development of specific preventive treatment includes those families in which the hearing is normal or near-normal at birth and then deteriorates rapidly in late infancy or childhood (9). At this time, not enough is known about the pathogenesis or even the histologic findings of the disease to permit treatment development.

A final form of preventive treatment that should be mentioned is prenatal diagnosis. In the past, the genetic counselor could only inform the parents of an affected child what their risk of recurrence was, and help them decide whether or not to have more children of their own, to adopt, or to utilize artificial insemination. However, it is now possible to diagnose an increasing number of genetic diseases prenatally by means of amniocentesis or other procedures. For couples who are willing to terminate the pregnancy if an abnormality is found, this option provides a way in which they can complete their families without the fear of a recurrence of the genetic abnormality. With rare exceptions, it is not possible at present to diagnose specific deafness syndromes prenatally. However, this is an area of very active research, and it seems likely that additional approaches to prenatal diagnosis will be developed in the near future.

To help prevent or treat deafness, an important job of the geneticist is to estimate the proportion of all cases of deafness that are genetically determined. It might seem that the easiest way to do this would be simply to count all of the families in which there were more than one affected child or an affected child and parent. However, this approach would fail to count as genetic all of the cases of recessive deafness in which, by chance, there was only one affected child in the family. As we have seen previously, recessive inheritance is the most common pattern of transmission and human families are so small that, in many families with recessive deafness, there is only one affected child. This approach would therefore lead to an underestimate of the proportion of genetic cases. The process by which we measure the true proportion of genetic cases can be likened to trying to estimate the size of an iceberg. If we know the relative density of ice and water, as well as the size of the part above the water, we can calculate the size of the entire iceberg. In a similar manner, if we know the proportion of families with more than one affected child and the distribution of affected children within those families, we can estimate what proportion of the families with only one affected child are actually genetic cases in which, by chance, only one child is deaf. When we applied this type of analysis to the large number of family histories of deaf couples that were collected by E.A. Fay in 1898, the overall estimate of the proportion of genetic cases turned out to be 54.9% with 45.1% being ascribed to nongenetic causes (12, 11). Somewhat surprisingly, when a similar estimate was obtained from family histories in a national survey collected by the Office of Demographic Studies at Gallaudet College in 1969 on more than 12,000 deaf children, the estimate was 50.7% genetic and 49.3% nongenetic (1).

One might have expected a decrease, rather than an increase in the proportion of nongenetic cases during the past 70 years in view of the dramatic advances that have been made in the treatment of infections, the management of premature infants, and the prevention of rubella and the effects of Rh incompatibility. It is possible that the expected trend will emerge in later data, particularly since the widespread use of immunization to prevent rubella did not occur until after 1969. Another disturbing possibility is that new, nongenetic causes of deafness may have appeared to replace those that have been reduced by improvements in medical care. We know, for example, that certain diseases, such as paralytic polio, are virtually nonexistent in primitive societies and begin to appear only when hygenic standards improve to the point at which all infants are no longer exposed to the virus during early infancy, at a time when retained maternal antibodies prevent serious disease. For similar reasons it is possible that rubella deafness may not have been as serious a problem during the 19th century as it was during the first 70 years of this century. Certain drugs are another nongenetic cause of deafness that is clearly a by-product of modern technology. Changes in mating patterns during the past century may also have contributed to the apparent reduction in the proportion of genetic deafness. As social and geographic mobility have increased, population isolates have tended to break up, and the incidence of inbreeding has declined. These changes would be expected to reduce the incidence of recessive deafness, at least temporarily. In the two studies mentioned previously, the estimated frequency of dominant deafness actually increased slightly, from 6.6% of all cases in the Fay study to 7.3% in the National Survey of the Deaf, while frequency of recessive deafness declined from 48.3% to 43.4%. Among the index cases in the national survey, 5.3% had at least one deaf parent while in the Fay study only 3.8% had a deaf parent. Since the frequency of deaf offspring from these matings has not changed, these findings suggest that there has been a substantial increase in the average fertility of the deaf during the past 70 years, which may well be related to improved educational opportunities and socioeconomic status.

At the present time, few schools for the deaf have organized genetic counseling programs, The Clarke School for the Deaf being a conspicuous exception to this generalization. In a recent institutional survey conducted by the Office of Demographic Studies at Gallaudet College, questionnaires were sent to 1,020 special educational programs for hearing impaired children. Of 421 programs that responded to the question "Does your program provide genetic counseling for your students and their families?" 49 or 11.6% answered affirmatively. Of the 49 positive responses, 11 were from residential schools for the deaf, 12 from day-school programs, and 26 from day-class programs (7). In a recent survey of the parents of students at Gallaudet College, only 7.4% identified the cause of deafness as being hereditary, although in 58.5% of the students a genetic etiology was readily apparent from the family history (7). Even in families where both parents and all the siblings were affected, only 14% were stated to be hereditary. It seems evident from these data that there is a major unmet need for genetic counseling of the deaf and for the parents of the deaf.

The process of genetic counseling has been extensively studied in hearing patients, but little is known about the factors which contribute to successful genetic counseling among the deaf. Most geneticists strongly support the view that the role of the genetic counselor should be to provide accurate genetic information to their clients in a nondirective manner, and to help them arrive at informed decisions that are consistent with their own beliefs and wishes. Cynics often argue that genetic counseling is never completely nondirective, and it is usually less so whenever it is necessary to over-simplify the intricacies of inheritance because of the level of understanding or educational background of the counselee. Thus a truly successful program for the provision of genetic counseling for the deaf should begin with a redesigning of the high school science curriculum, to be sure that it includes an adequate coverage of the principles of human genetics.

As mentioned previously, one of the most difficult problems in counseling families with hereditary deafness is attempting to distinguish between nongenetic deafness and cases of recessive deafness in which there are no other close relatives who are affected. Many parents are unable to provide accurate information on third- and fourth-degree relatives and it is possible that, if more complete pedigrees were available, the hereditary nature of additional cases would become apparent. To test this hypothesis, the author conducted a study of the student body of Gallaudet College during the 1973-1974 school year to determine how often remote genealogic relationships could be established among the deaf (8). A total of 812 questionnaires requesting detailed family history data were sent to the parents of students of the college. Of these, 555 usable forms were returned, containing information on a total of more than 10,000 individuals. Seventy-seven percent of the students were estimated to have genetic deafness of whom 24% had dominant and 76% recessive deafness. The collected pedigree data were then matched against the roster of some 30,000 individuals in families of the deaf that had been collected by E.A. Fay in 1898. The parents of 322 Gallaudet students were able to provide pedigree data on one or more ancestors who were born in this country before 1900. Of these, there were certain or possible pedigree linkages with the Fay data in 18 records or 7.3% of the genetic cases. This experience gave evidence that the establishment of genealogic linkages through a national registry of hereditary deafness would serve a valuable function in identifying cases of hereditary deafness. In order to search the registry, a user would have to supply pedigree data that would contribute to the file, and thus the effectiveness of the registry would increase the more it is used. A deafness registry could have many other useful purposes. It could lead to the identification of groups of individuals who, by genetic criteria, have the same form of hereditary deafness. A major goal of research in clinical genetics during the next decade will be to determine the chromosomal location of genes for specific hereditary syndromes. In the case of hereditary deafness, not a single syndrome has yet been "mapped" except for those known to be caused by genes carried on the X chromosome. The identification of large kinships of affected individuals who would be interested in participating in this research effort, would greatly facilitate the chromosomal mapping of human genes for deafness. In a similar manner, many other kinds of clinical, psychological, and educational research and services might profit greatly from the identification of groups of individuals who have the same type of deafness. Finally, it should be noted that the establishment of genealogic linkages as a method for identifying cases of hereditary deafness is not a new or radical idea. As long ago as 1883, Alexander Graham Bell, whose interest in hereditary deafness is well known, became impressed by the frequent recurrence of unusual surnames among the rosters of schools for the deaf. "The inference is irresistable," Bell concluded, "that in many cases the recurrences indicated blood relationships among the pupils." With the advent of modern computer technology, the establishment of a national registry of hereditary deafness may be an idea whose time has come.

Note: This is paper number 13 from the Department of Human Genetics of the Medical College of Virginia and was supported in part by grant #C-178 from the National Foundation. I gratefully acknowledge the assistance of Ms. Phyllis Winter and Mrs. Patricia Fox in the preparation of this manuscript.

3

Lyle L. Lloyd, Ph.D. and
Arthur J. Dahle, Ph.D.

Detection and Diagnosis
Of a Hearing Impairment in the Child

Dr. Lloyd is health scientist administrator for communication disorders at the Mental Retardation Branch of the National Institute of Child Health and Human Development, the National Institutes of Health, Bethesda, Maryland.

Dr. Dahle is director of the speech and hearing division at the Center of Development and Learning Disorders, University of Alabama, Birmingham.

Recent audiologic developments in areas of detection and diagnosis represent the efforts of numerous professionals dedicated to finding more efficient and reliable approaches to assessing the functioning of the auditory mechanism. New techniques have been developed to evaluate the auditory system at various points from the middle ear to the cortex. Research has focused on improving both behavioral and electrophysiologic procedures and, with few exceptions, the current developments represent refinements of technology and procedures that have been in existence for many years. Perhaps this trend represents a certain level of professional maturity wherein new advances evolve naturally in the course of ever-expanding knowledge.

As with all new scientific and clinical developments, acceptance of new audiologic techniques by professionals and consumers must stand the test of time and practical application. Clinical procedures which emerged during the past decade are no exception, and some have fallen short of expectations while others show signs of becoming well established.

To a significant extent, most of the new developments have centered around materials, instrumentation, and techniques for evaluating young children and other difficult-to-test populations; a trend encouraging to those faced with the difficult task of early detection and diagnosis of auditory impairments. This chapter will focus primarily on the developments in the area of pediatric audiology; it is divided into four partially overlapping sections covering a) hearing screening and early identification, b) behavioral audiometry, c) speech audiometry, and d) electrophysiologic procedures.

Hearing Screening and Early Identification

The realization that language and auditory skills are most effectively developed during the first few years of life has served as a major motivation for developing procedures for detecting hearing impairments in infants. Many investigators during the early 1960's reported on techniques for assessing hearing sensitivity in newborns and young infants that relied on eliciting behavioral responses to various auditory stimuli (45, 47, 182, 42). These procedures, based on the early work of the Ewings', have frequently been referred to as behavior observation audiometry (BOA) (69). Although Hardy, Dougherty, and Hardy (84) were among the first to use this technique on a large scale, Downs and Sterritt (50) provided the first evidence that mass hearing screening of newborns could be conducted by volunteers in hospitals on a routine basis. The pioneering work by Downs and her colleagues in the early 1960's served as a catalyst for generating interest in infant hearing testing, which subsequently led to the establishment of newborn hearing-screening programs in several hospitals across the nation. However, clinical experience with the procedure soon revealed that behavior observation screening resulted in unacceptably high percentages of false-positives which, along with other methodological problems, served to reduce confidence in the feasibility of screening infants on a routine basis. Eisenberg (56) served to focus attention on these problems by identifying potential sources for error in studying neonatal behavior which included the stimuli, the organism's response, and the accuracy of detecting responses. Moncur (137) and Ling, Ling, and Doehring (111) also identified difficulties in obtaining observer accuracy and agreement in judging infant responses to sound, although Weber (179, 180) demonstrated that accuracy of observation could be improved through careful structuring of the procedures for observing and recording responses. Other attempts to improve screening procedures included modification of the test stimuli (160), using both a broad band signal and pure tone to help differentiate between hearing impairment and general inattentiveness to sound. In spite of improvements in test procedures, problems were encountered in conducting mass infant hearing-screening programs which eventually led to a reassessment of the efficacy and economy of screening on a routine basis (79, 72, 48), and critiques stressed that neonatal hearing screening did not accomplish its objectives and failed to identify many children with less severe losses and/or progressive impairments.

The questions raised concerning neonatal screening led to the establishment of the AAOO-AAP-ASHA* Joint Committee on Infant Hearing Screening. The Committee's report (1) discouraged routine hearing screening for newborns which was not research oriented. A supplementary statement of the Joint Committee (2) recommended that infants at high risk for hearing impairment should be identified by means of history and physical examination. Risk factors consisted of: a history of hereditary childhood hearing impairment; rubella or other nonbacterial intrauterine fetal infection; defects of ear, nose, and throat; birth weight less than 1500 grams; and/or bilirubin level greater than 20 mg/100 ml serum. Children identified as being high risk on one or more factors were recommended for referral for in-depth audiologic evaluation during their first two months of life and follow-up hearing

---

*American Association of Otolaryngology and Ophthalmology-American Association of Pediatrics-American Speech and Hearing Association.

evaluations in a physician's office or well-baby clinics. The Conference on Newborn Hearing Screening held in San Francisco (34) made similar recommendations for using a registry for identifying newborns who are high-risk for hearing impairment. Based on this approach, the "A.B.C.D.'s" to H.E.A.R. was published (49). This mnemonic device is designed to help physicians remember the principal risk factors to be considered. High-risk indicators in the newborn nursery were listed as: *A*ffected family; *B*ilirubin level…; *C*ongenital rubella syndrome; *D*efects of the ear, nose, or throat; and *S*mall at birth. They went on to list items to be assessed in subsequent visits as: *H*earing concern? *E*ar test normal? *A*waken to sound? *R*esponses in the developmental and communication scale?

However, on the basis of more current research, the use of a high-risk registry in conjunction with neonatal hearing-screening is recommended (129, 130, 173). Although research results show a higher prevalence of confirmed deafness for the high-risk groups, it has been found that hearing-screening identified some children who would have been missed by the high-risk registry. Investigators recommend testing hearing by eliciting an arousal response during light sleep. Based on the combined approach, a comprehensive set of guidelines (148) for identifying deafness in infants has been presented that includes detailed suggestions for applying a high-risk registry, screening hearing, conducting follow-up audiologic evaluations, and monitoring the hearing of infants at a physician's office or clinic.

On the basis of recent research, the current emphasis placed on the use of high-risk factors in identifying children who may be susceptible to hearing impairments appears to be well founded. For example, a high prevalence of sensorineural hearing impairment in a group of 3- to 6-year-olds with subclinical or inapparent congenital cytomegalovirus infection has been reported (156, 37). These children had no observable symptoms and normally would not have been seen for hearing evaluations, except for the presence of the high-risk factor of intrauterine viral infection. Peckham (150) demonstrated that many children with congenital rubella may develop hearing impairments which are not manifested at birth; this suggests that the use of a high-risk registry would aid in identifying children with progressive hearing loss who might otherwise go undetected.

During the last decade, identification audiometry for older children has received less attention in the literature since procedures were well established during the 1950's. The most current ASHA statements on school-age identification audiometry (4) are similar to the earlier guidelines (40). Both reports recommended testing children individually, using discrete frequency air conduction pure tone procedures. Current guidelines recommend screening at 1000 Hz, 2000 Hz, and 4000 Hz in typical school settings. The addition of 500 Hz is also desirable when testing is conducted in better acoustic environments. Although the ASHA Guidelines specify testing with pure tones, some interest has been generated in the past 10 years in the use of the Verbal Auditory Screening for Children (VASC) Test (81). Although the VASC has been reported to be useful for screening hearing of young children with normal intelligence (86, 82) and retarded children (39), other investigators have raised questions concerning the accuracy of the VASC test in identifying children with mild hearing losses (157), high-frequency impairments (32), and conductive pathology (35). Consequently, pure-tone screening procedures continue to be the method of choice since they reduce the possibility of overlooking children with significant hearing impairments. A more recent research report on the VASC and other identification audiometry procedures is in general support of the previous reports (71).

Projections: Comprehensive research on early auditory behavior should lead to improvements in assessing the hearing of infants (57). To become practical, however, mass hearing screening for newborns will probably be based on automated programs that reduce reliance on trained personnel and observer judgment. Such a procedure has been developed by using a "Crib-o-gram" program that automatically monitors the responses of several infants by means of motion-sensitive transducers attached to isolettes (169). Preliminary data indicate that the technique is at least as valid and efficient as the use of human observers and has the potential for much greater accuracy through the use of computer scoring of responses. Similar to the findings of other investigators, test accuracy was found to be best when babies were tested during regular or light sleep. The use of high-risk registries will necessitate considerably more testing of infants in audiology centers, and refinement of operant audiometry (120) and impedance audiometry (101, 21, 127) for use with infants and children should find increased application in future audiologic follow-up programs. Use of sucking response pattern changes to pure tones also holds much promise as a potential method for screening the hearing of infants (55).

Continued research on high-risk factors should also help expand our capability for early identification of hearing impaired children. Studies previously cited involving longitudinal work with rubella and cytomegalovirus along with other infectious agents hopefully will lead to improved methods of identifying and monitoring high-risk children (102, 83, 110). Research on genetic and metabolic causes of deafness should also aid in identifying the hearing impaired at an early age. However, probably the most important goal for the future is to develop comprehensive systems for early detection, management, and treatment of the hearing impaired involving organization of many agencies and professionals for following an infant from birth through childhood. At present, only a very few communities have hearing-screening programs for children under 2 or 3 years of age and in general, health delivery in this country is highly fragmented. To capitalize on available resources, Lloyd has proposed screening hearing in conjunction with the normal immunization sequence routinely administered to infants at 2, 4, 6, 12, and 18 months (117). He suggested follow-up testing of all high-risk infants at all five age levels with routine hearing screening of all infants at the 4-, 6-, 12-, and 18-month immunization visits. As the technology to implement comprehensive identification programs already exists, it would appear that the greatest challenge for the future will be to convince the public and other health professionals of the need and feasibility of detecting hearing impairment in infancy.

Behavioral Audiometry

Behavioral audiometry is a general term used to describe audiometric procedures that are designed to use operant response to sound. Basically the examiner's task is to bring operant behavior (voluntary, controlled, and/or conditioned responses) under stimulus control (115). Although operant conditioning is sometimes restricted to mean those situations which utilize structured reinforcement schedules, it has been pointed out that all behavioral audiometric tests can be viewed as an operant procedure (114). Operant behavior is differentiated from respondent (involuntary, reflexive, or physiologic) behavior on the basis of the stimulus-response relationship. Respondents are influenced or controlled primarily by the antecedent stimulus while operants are influenced by events or consequences, e.g., reinforcement, which immediately follow the response (115). Thus, in behavioral audiometry, the test stimulus may have little or no effect on a subject's behavior without careful consideration of the reinforcing stimuli that occur immediately following the response. Therefore, in behavioral audiometry the subject's response and the contingent reinforcement are extremely critical variables.

In view of the ability to control or modify operant behavior with reinforcement, it is not surprising that most of the early work in behavioral audiometry with children focused attention on the use of various reinforcers. Conditioned play audiometry utilizes social reinforcement in conjunction with subject participation in an "interesting" play activity (93, 5, 63). This technique has been shown to result in threshold measures which are essentially equivalent to standard procedures (122, 119). Pioneering studies have produced novel types of visually reinforcing consequences, and include procedures such as the Peep Show, Slide Show, Pup Show, COR, CAVRA, and the Toy Train Test (58, 46, 174, 149, 112). Initially, response parameters did not receive as much consideration as the reinforcer, and the behavior required of the subject varied from button pushing to head-turn localization.

It was not until the early 1960's that researchers investigated the use of tangible reinforcers in a strict operant conditioning paradigm to find a way of testing low-functioning retarded individuals (104, 132, 133, 171, 16, 17, 193, 67). The outgrowth of work with the retarded led to the development of a procedure that is commonly called Tangible Reinforcement Operant Conditioning Audiometry (TROCA) (121). Although TROCA was originally designed for testing the hearing of the nonverbal, severely retarded, the procedure was also shown to be applicable to evaluating normal infants by successfully testing three 7- to 18-month-old infants (121). The extension of operant conditioning audiometry to nonretarded infants and young children has recently been shown to be a powerful technique for the determination of pure-tone thresholds in children as young as 7 to 8 months of age (120, 188, 187). In addition to the refinement of TROCA techniques for use with infants, the use of visual reinforcers has also recently been refined for more effective use with very young children (138, 188, 139, 189). Investigators demonstrated that threshold responses could be elicited in infants as young as 4 months of age by the careful application of visual reinforcers. The use of visual reinforcers in conjunction with a head-turn localization response has often been referred to as "Conditioned Orientation Reflex" (COR) audiometry, a term stemming from early work in which the localization response was thought to be an orienting reflex (174). Most clinicians now feel the term is misleading, as at least for older children the response is an operant rather than a respondent, i.e., reflective. Visual reinforcement audiometry (VRA) or conditioned orientation response (COR) audiometry would appear to be more appropriate labels for this procedure. In any event, the careful, controlled use of visual reinforcers is a relatively effective approach that requires less sophisticated instrumentation than TROCA.

Behavior observation audiometry (BOA) is another commonly used behavioral procedure which relies on the observation of overt behavioral response to the occurrence of sound* (142, 118, 8, 31, 69, 109, 116). Careful application of a BOA procedure has been shown to produce valuable information when used with young children (177); however, most research and clinical experience has demonstrated that TROCA and visual reinforcement audiometry result in more reliable and valid threshold responses (187, 189). For more in-depth information on behavioral audiometry the reader is encouraged to read the text by Fulton and Lloyd (69).

Projections: Although the effectiveness of TROCA in obtaining threshold measures was well documented almost a decade ago, many clinicians continue to rely solely on behavior observation audiometry for evaluating young children. Hopefully, recent improvements in instrumentation and procedures will result in increased use of both TROCA and visual reinforcement audiometry. The use of operant conditioning in testing infants should also become a more routine proce-

---

*BOA may use operant and/or respondent behavior. However, it primarily involves operant responses—the exception being its use with young infants.

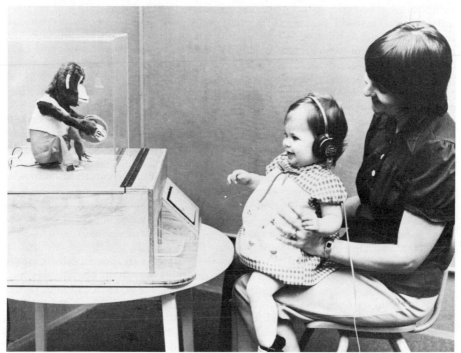

This 12-month-old girl has just pushed a button on hearing an auditory stimulus and is enjoying visual reinforcement, an animated toy monkey. Taken from a project conducted by Dr. Wesley R. Wilson, University of Washington Child Development and Mental Retardation Center, Seattle. Photo Courtesy of Jan Smyth, CDMRC Media Service.

dure for both early detection and diagnosis of auditory impairments. Recent applications of operant principles to site-of-lesion testing (67) and speech discrimination testing (36, 188, 52) can be expected to lead to techniques for extending special auditory diagnostic procedures to much younger age levels. The value of behavioral procedures lies in their wide range of application, and future developments in this area should provide the technology for evaluating almost all auditory functions regardless of the individual's age or intellectual level. The extensive work being conducted using a sucking response to measure audition in very young infants, and more recently the use of the head-turn response to assess the speech discrimination of infants, is evidence of how far we have progressed during the past decade and serves as an indicator of future directions in behavioral audiometry (54, 26, 25, 53, 141, 55, 188, 52).

Speech Audiometry

Although several auditory functions can be assessed to describe an individual's ability to hear speech, most clinicians continue to rely on only two measures: the threshold of intelligibility of spondaic words and the discrimination of "phonetically balanced" (PB) monosyllabic words at supra-threshold levels. The persistence in the use of these procedures is quite remarkable considering that most of our traditional speech reception tests evolved from work conducted decades ago at Bell

Telephone Laboratories (60), Harvard Psychoacoustic Laboratory (51), and the Central Institute for the Deaf (88). Although the use of spondaic words for speech-threshold testing continues to be the stimulus of choice for most clinicians, the reliance on use of phonetically balanced word lists has been questioned by a number of investigators (27, 176, 28). There have been attempts to develop alternative measures of speech intelligibility for adults such as the Rhyme Test (59), the Modified Rhyme Test (91), and synthetic sentences (170), but these procedures are not routinely used in most clinics.

The standard speech-audiometric tests were developed for adults and require echoic or written responses that often limit their use for evaluating children. Even the controlled vocabulary PB word lists (87, 92) are not suitable for use with the very young child or children with speech and language impairments. Special considerations are needed in conducting auditory measurements with children in relation to stimulus materials, response mode, instructional modes, and motivational factors (64). Based on consideration of these factors, several speech hearing tests have been designed specifically for use with children; some sought to avoid the need for a verbal response by developing picture tests of speech discrimination (143, 144). The Threshold by Identification of Pictures (TIP) and the Discrimination by Identification of Pictures (DIP) tests were developed to assess both threshold and supra-threshold discrimination of speech in children (168). The DIP test was designed to measure speech discrimination on the basis of acoustic phonetic factors and is normed for use with children as young as 3 years of age. The Word Intelligibility by Picture Identification (WIPI) test (161) is also normed for use with young children. In addition to auditory discrimination, this test can be used to assess visual and combined auditory-visual discrimination. The WIPI has another advantage over most other picture-response tests in that it has several equivalent forms and a larger number of foil items that serve to reduce the effect of guessing. The G-F-W Test of Auditory Discrimination (73) and the G-F-W Diagnostic Auditory Discrimination Test (75) are picture-tests normed for a wide age range. Although these test instruments were not designed specifically for use with the hearing impaired, their provisions for pretraining and item error analysis indicate great potential for use in the audiologic assessment of young children.

A factor sometimes overlooked by audiologists is that performance on speech discrimination tests may vary considerably depending upon test construction and mode of response (146, 106, 113, 119). Thus, the clinician cannot assume that performance on a closed-set picture response test will be equivalent to scores made on an open-set echoic response test. The question of which technique provides the most valid information is open to debate; however, the choice of procedure will most often be dictated by the needs of the client.

The Wepman Auditory Discrimination Test (183), which requires a same-different response to pairs of words, has been primarily used in studying children with speech impairments and/or learning disabilities. The unfamiliar vocabulary, and the use of the terms "same" and "different," and the reliance on a verbal response make it difficult to use this test with young children. A paired comparison test of auditory discrimination, in which the child is asked to point to the pair of pictures that have been named, avoids the need for a verbal response or the use of the terms "same" or "different" (154). In general, however, speech sound (or word) discrimination results obtained with same-different or paired comparison procedures may be influenced by attention, vocabulary, and other factors, making their use as a routine test of discrimination questionable (12).

Among the several specialized adaptations of speech-hearing tests devised during the past few years are the dichotic listening tests (11, 100). These tests, along with other specialized measures (89), are designed to measure higher-level auditory functions and can be used to assist in identifying impairments in the central auditory pathways. Specialized auditory perceptual tests have also been developed specifically for use with children. The Goldman-Fristoe-Woodcock Auditory Skills Test Battery (1974) contains 12 tests designed to assess a wide range of auditory functions including discrimination, selective attention, memory, phonemic synthesis, sequencing, and sound-symbol association. The G-F-W test battery, along with other tests of auditory perception, certainly holds potential for measuring higher-level auditory functioning of the hearing impaired (99, 184, 185, 191, 23, 22, 66, 128, 61, 62). For example, it would appear important to measure such functions as auditory memory and sequencing in the hearing impaired to provide information for planning individualized auditory training and language remediation programs. A recently compiled guide to available language intervention programs includes information on several auditory perceptual programs (65).

Projections: Recent applications of operant procedures to speech discrimination testing indicate potential for applying operant conditioning principles to speech-hearing tests for the evaluation of young children and other difficult-to-test subjects (36, 188, 52). The recent development of speech perception tests should encourage further development and application of diagnostic speech-hearing tests and structured instructional programs for remediation of deficits (184, 185, 191, 23, 66, 75, 128, 61, 62). Research conducted with infants has demonstrated that many speech-hearing skills are developed very early in life (135, 178, 25, 53, 141). Also, there is recent evidence that research techniques for assessing speech perception in infants may soon find application in clinical use (188, 52). This work in evaluating speech discrimination through adaptation of visual reinforcement audiometric techniques indicates the feasibility of assessing speech discrimination in a clinical setting in infants as young as 6 months of age. Thus, these investigators have shown that the assessment of speech-hearing functions in children is limited only by our ability to apply the principles involved in controlling and modifying operant and respondent behavior.

Electrophysiologic Procedures

The neurophysiology of the auditory mechanism provides many avenues for eliciting respondent responses to auditory stimulation. Therefore, it is not surprising that several neurophysiologic or electrophysiologic measures have been developed to elicit responses to sound mediated by the peripheral and central nervous system.

Hogan (90) lists the functional activities of the heart, sweat glands, eyes, and lungs as the most potentially useful autonomic nervous system (ANS) responses to auditory stimulation. Electrodermal or galvanic skin responses are thought to be mediated by the action of sweat glands in relation to changes in an individual's emotional state. Audiometric parameters related to electrodermal responses have been studied extensively (76), and procedures based on this phenomenon have found clinical application in evaluation of individuals with suspected functional hearing impairments (145). Although some papers in the 1950's proposed that electrodermal response (EDR) audiometry was useful in evaluating young children and the retarded (85, 5, 94, 105), later reports identified many methodologic and humanistic problems that contraindicate its use with most difficult-to-test children (149, 103, 115). Currently, the primary use of electrodermal audiometry is in evaluating compensation cases for the Veterans Administration (103).

Changes in heart rate in response to auditory stimulation have been well documented for adults (194), infants (6, 7, 167), and older children (166). The nature of the cardiac response to sound appears to vary with maturation. Neonates tend to exhibit cardiac acceleration (6), while infants over 4 months of age show deceleration (29). Evaluation of the procedure indicates that heart rate can be used successfully as a response to auditory signals (7, 172). Comparison with electroencephalographic responses suggests that both heart rate and related vascular responses may be more sensitive and less subject to error (166, 38). However, heart rate audiometry was not found to be successful with mentally retarded persons (24) and further research will be needed to standardize test methodology and validate its use with different populations.

Respiration audiometry has also generated much interest since the 1960's as a method for assessing hearing sensitivity. One of the first studies to employ respiration rate audiometry found that respiration rates did not change when auditory stimuli were presented to deaf children, but did change when stimuli were presented to normals and subjects with milder losses (159). Recently, results were reported for a series of studies in which only 15% of 498 ears tested by respiration and behavioral audiometry resulted in a difference of more than ± 15dB between the two methods (14). There is a suggestion that it is a valid technique for obtaining pure-tone thresholds in children and adults and can be used as a routine clinical tool for assessing difficult-to-test patients (15). In view of the most recent research, respiration audiometry must be considered as a potential clinical procedure for the detection and diagnosis of hearing impairment.

However, the results from studies reporting that respiration audiometry may result in differences as large as 15dB from behavioral thresholds suggest caution in interpreting results from this procedure. It has been stressed that too little is known about autonomic nervous system responses to recommend them for general clinical usage (90). Thus, it would appear that more research is needed to validate the clinical application of all respondent procedures involving ANS responses.

It has been known for many years that changes in the electrical activity of the brain may be elicited or evoked through stimulation by an auditory signal (41). The electroencephalographic (EEG) response to sound has been utilized by many investigators as a measure of hearing sensitivity. Early attempts to detect EEG responses to acoustic stimuli (190, 134) were cumbersome and difficult to interpret. Although the advent of the average response computer provided a much more reliable approach to measuring cortical evoked responses (80, 43, 125, 123), many methodological problems render it impractical for routine clinical use (153). Evoked Response Audiometry (ERA) or, as some prefer, Averaged Evoked Response (AER) audiometry, has generally focused on the late (50-400 msec) response components, which are thought to reflect cortical activity. Reports on the middle (10 - 50 msec) latency response components (78, 77) and the early* (less than 10 msec latency) brainstem potentials (152, 70) appear to hold much greater promise for use in assessing auditory sensitivity. In particular, wave V of the early components has been found to be a relatively consistent response which is resistant to many of the physiological factors that affect the late responses (98, 70).

Electrocochleography is a direct measurement of the functioning of the cochlea. This procedure has been of interest to researchers since the presence of cochlear microphonics that originate in the hair cells of the organ of Corti was identified

---

*It should be noted that previously many individuals referred to 10-50 mesc latency as the early components.

(186). The addition of the identification of the action potentials of the auditory nerve provided the basis for most current electrocochleography (ECoG) procedures (44). Interest in applying electrocochleography as a clinical procedure was generated by reports of measuring cochlear potentials and eighth nerve action potentials from electrodes placed near the round window in patients undergoing ear surgery (164, 163, 162). However, more current work, using signal averaging, indicates that action potentials with latencies of 2 - 3 msec can be measured reliably through placement of the electrode in the outer ear canal (33, 10). The use of a nonsurgical procedure certainly enhances the possibility for greater clinical application. Nevertheless, the need to restrict the patient's physical activity will probably prevent its use for young children in most clinical settings. In this respect, the procedure is similar to GSR audiometry in that it is most difficult to use with the individuals who have the greatest need for its use.

The introduction of impedance audiometry as a clinical tool is one of the most noteworthy audiologic developments to occur during the past decade. Seldom has a new procedure gained such wide acceptance and use in such a short span of time. Although impedance audiometry has been employed in Europe for a number of years, it was only during the late 1960's and early 1970's that the procedure began to be widely used in this country. During this interval, impedance audiometry has become a routine part of most audiologic evaluations.

The first clinically useful impedance audiometric procedure was developed by Metz (131) using an electromechanical method for measuring relative changes in acoustic impedance in the middle ear. Although Zwislocki later continued to use an electromechanical bridge to measure absolute impedance of the middle ear, current impedance audiometric procedures are based on electroacoustic methods of measurement. The early research on impedance audiometry, conducted primarily in Scandinavian countries, provided the basic technology and experience necessary for development as a clinical tool. Other important contributions provided clinical validation of the usefulness of impedance audiometry in the routine evaluation of the hearing of both children and adults (19, 3, 95).

Although the physical basis of impedance measurement is fairly complex (9), the clinical application is relatively simple and can be completed in a very short period of time by an experienced clinician. Basic impedance audiometry includes at least three separate types of measurements consisting of tympanometry, static compliance, and stapedius reflex thresholds. Although both tympanometry and static compliance measure the compliance or mobility of the middle ear system, tympanometry is thought to provide more reliable information. The stapedius reflex provides information on cochlear functioning through determination of the threshold at which pure tones cause the stapedial muscle to contract.

The capability of using a respondent procedure to measure middle ear functioning and, to some degree, the integrity of the sensorineural mechanism, holds great potential for use with very young children and other difficult-to-test individuals. Verification of impedance audiometry with children has indeed demonstrated that it is a valuable technique for evaluating infants and young children (18, 20, 158, 13, 97). The procedure has been shown to be valid for use even with newborns (101), and impedance audiometry is also reported to be used effectively with retarded subjects (107, 108, 68).

Although impedance audiometry is normally used as part of a test battery in a comprehensive evaluation, it has been found to have potential for use as a screening device also (21, 127). However, its use as a screening instrument raises an interesting question of what constitutes identifiable pathology, since tympanometry may be more sensitive in the detection of ear pathology than visual inspection of the middle ear by an otolaryngologist (148). Also, impedance audiometry cannot be relied on to detect sensorineural hearing loss and thus cannot be substituted for pure tone audiometry as a screening procedure (13).

In addition to the basic measurements, impedance audiometry has many other potential uses. Its use in making gross predictions of degree and slope of hearing loss has been reported (97). Jerger's procedure, based on the work of Niemeyer and Sesterhenn (147), measures the difference between acoustic reflex thresholds for pure tones and broad band noise. In evaluating this procedure on a large number of patients, Jerger found no errors in prediction of general sensitivity categories (grossly normal, mild-moderate loss, severe loss, or profound loss) in 60% of the cases; serious errors (difference of two or more categories) were found in only 4% of the ears tested. Jerger (96) also suggested other intriguing diagnostic uses, such as measuring loudness recruitment and reflex decay. Recent advances in instrumentation, e.g., ipsilateral reflex testing, serve to extend the usefulness of impedance audiometry and its possible use in hearing aid evaluation with young children and justify optimism that impedance audiometry will continue to generate interest for both researchers and clinicians (126).

Projections: The clinician's insatiable quest for evaluating all levels of the auditory system assures the continued development and refinement of electrophysiologic audiometric procedures. Certainly the use and refinement of impedance audiometry will continue for many years. The future should also see increased application of nonsurgical electrocochleography and measurement of very early components of cortical evoked potentials (98, 152). An intriguing future use of cortically evoked potentials lies in their application for evaluation of higher-level auditory perceptual functions (181, 155) and cerebral dominance (30, 124, 140, 165, 192, 136, 151, 175). These developments should be of particular importance to assessing auditory and language functioning in infants and other difficult-to-test individuals. Continued research on the use of ANS auditory response measures may also facilitate their application in detecting and diagnosing hearing impairments. In particular, the use of heart rate and respiration audiometric procedures should become more common as methods are standardized and validated. Certainly, electrophysiologic audiometric procedures based on respondent behavior can be expected to play an increasingly important role in the future. However, it must be remembered that respondents cannot measure how or what one "hears"; they can only be used to reveal the integrity of the auditory system. Nevertheless, the ability to detect and measure the transmission of auditory signals at precise points in pathways can be of tremendous importance in diagnosing the location and cause of hearing impairment.

The next decade should see many new developments for detecting and diagnosing hearing impairments. One can only guess what course these new procedures will follow, but it seems safe to speculate that they will focus on the evaluation of infants and multiply-handicapped children. Hopefully, continued research on the nature of normal auditory development will provide a basis for designing more sophisticated procedures, not only for diagnosing impairments, but for evaluating developmental lags and prescribing remediation strategies.

4

Edna S. Levine, Ph.D.

Psychological Contributions

Dr. Levine is professor emeritus, New York University, New York City.

In certain respects, psychology and the deaf appear to share a common problem: both labor under a stereotypic image of limited operational resources. In the case of psychology, the stereotype is narrowed to only a few of the profession's better known operations. Testing is an example. Less familiar but equally, if not more, important functions generally go unrecognized.

In the review that follows of psychology's contributions over the past decade, examples are given to illustrate both sorts of functions, the familiar and the less familiar. These include: a) self-study; b) advocacy and outreach; c) training; d) service; and e) research.

Self-Study

The success or failure of psychological services rests with the competencies of the service provider. This being so, periodic self-study to maintain professional standards of competance is an essential function of psychology. In view of the broadened services for deaf persons, it becomes a professional imperative for psychology to put its own house in order in regard to this population, to cast a critical eye on its practices and problems, and take whatever steps are necessary to serve the deaf with competence.

A project specifically designed to meet this imperative was a contribution of the period under review. The self-study approach took the form of a comprehensive questionnaire-survey of the backgrounds, preparation, practices, and problems of a national sampling of 178 psychological service providers to the deaf operating in a variety of settings (46). The findings disclosed a depressing picture of the inferred quality of psychological services. Among other handicaps, the large majority of respondents were practicing without in-depth knowledge of deafness and the deaf, without special preparation for their work, and without the ability to communicate manually or to establish productive interpersonal relations with their manual clients. Problems were further compounded by exceptional difficulties in the use

23

and interpretation of psychological tests with the deaf. The urgent recommendation of the respondents was for follow-up conferences.

The recommendation was swiftly carried out in the form of a national conference (the Spartanburg Conference) of providers and multidisciplinary consumers of psychological services for the deaf. Among its major achievements were clear delineations of the functions and competencies expected of psychologists to the deaf, and drafts of possible training strategies whereby the necessary competencies could be acquired. A further conference is in planning at which these delineations will be used as guides in structuring proposed training programs and in setting up standards for the qualification of psychologists to the deaf and for the accreditation of training programs for these workers. The anticipated outcome of these endeavors is to produce psychologists who are able to serve the deaf with excellence and accountability.

Advocacy and Outreach

A psychologist's responsibility to a deaf client does not end with preparing the individual to make his way into hearing society. This is only one side of the service coin. The other involves preparing society to receive the deaf person, hopefully with understanding and insight. Unless this can be accomplished, a psychologist's labors are in danger of being hopelessly undone by society's ignorance and indifference. Advocacy and outreach are, therefore, highly important psychological functions. The following are illustrations of how two psychologists conducted their respective advocacy-outreach functions in behalf of the deaf in the period under review.

First is the campaign conducted by McCay Vernon, directed not only to public and professional circles but more spectacularly to the traditional bastion of deaf persons themselves—the educational establishment. Impelled by passionate indignation with the wasted human potential in the deaf population, and with education's failures in developing these potentials (2, 80), Vernon, among other acts, disseminated the evidence of 50 years of psychological investigation asserting the normal mental potential of the deaf (81). He then went on to point the accusing finger at oralism as the factor he considered chiefly responsible for the poor showing of the deaf in scholastic and personal fulfillment. He espoused instead the use of total communication (see Garretson, chapter 13) both in the school and in the home.

To get his message across, Vernon employed all relevant psychological principles and techniques of persuasive mass communication and communicator credibility. That he succeeded in the task is by now a matter of record with increasing numbers of programs for the deaf adopting his recommendations and viewpoint.

It is an almost unheard of advocacy-achievement for psychology to pit itself against an entrenched educational system and make any sort of impact in the short span of a decade. But this has proved to be one of its more extraordinary accomplishments in the field of the deaf. The ultimate confirmation of Vernon's views will of course have to wait for time and research. But in the meantime, the sparks are flying. Hopefully, they will help light the dark in which education of the deaf has been groping for so long.

The second illustration of outreach is of quite different character both in regard to target and strategy. The principal incentive was the near-panic expressed in private communications to the psychologist-advocate by teachers and fellow-psychologists in the regular schools concerning the management of mainstreamed deaf children. Both they and their nondeaf pupils were at a loss. Next, was the deep frustration voiced by numbers of disability areas with the difficulties involved in improving ingrained negative attitudes of the adult public toward its disabled members (24). Another lead came from a searching investigation of attitudes toward the deaf which stressed the importance of knowledge about deafness as a key aid in effecting attitude change (56). The final and decision-making influence came from the old psychological adage that it is easier to form attitudes at the child level than to change ingrained attitudes at the adult level.

Combining the input from all these sources, the advocacy strategy took the form of an illustrated children's book for young hearing readers written by the psychologist-advocate to describe what deafness means, what it does, and how deaf children develop the unusual skills needed to overcome the handicaps (45). As with the Vernon strategy, it is too soon to judge the outcome of this approach, but the selection of the book by the Child Study Association of America, Inc. as among the best children's books of 1974 is promising. If the psychological adage previously cited holds true, it is possible that the understandings implanted at the child level will be retained through life as a pattern of acceptance and admiration toward persons who are deaf.

Training

The lack of programs to prepare psychologists for work with the deaf has been previously noted. Therefore, to fulfill their training function, the more experienced psychologists to the deaf have had to take a different route to reach their less experienced colleagues. A principal one of the past decade has been the production of an impressive number of guides, orientative materials, and special informational literature dealing with various aspects of psychological practice with the deaf.

A small sampling of references to such literature gives some indication of the scope covered, and, less directly, of the unmet training needs. Included among the publications are guides to: the psychological evaluation of deaf adults and clients (79, 83, 11, 12, 47), mental assessment of deaf children (44); techniques of counseling (27, 76, 13); behavior modification with the deaf (48); and problems and management of multihandicapped deaf children and adults (82, 9, 41).

Obviously, mass communicated "how-to-do-it-yourself" approaches to psychological practice cannot be condoned. But in the lack of organized training programs, the guides represent the principal training-lifeline for many inexperienced psychologists floundering about in the vaguely charted waters of psychological operations with the deaf.

Service

Included in this ruthlessly abridged digest of services is a special bow to the service providers who, without fuss or fanfare, go about their daily tasks of administering psychological first-aid as required, support for parents, and enlightenment for a wide variety of involved professionals from other disciplines. Such services include: evaluation and diagnosis; advisement and counseling; psychotherapeutic interventions; educational and vocational guidance; collaboration with community agencies; parent groups, legislative groups; inservice orientation; collaboration with other specialists; report writing; writing grant applications; crisis intervention; advocacy and outreach; plus all the multiple services subsumed under these general groupings. It is obvious even from this brief listing that service is the backbone function of psychological practice.

Research

Compared with previous periods (43) the past 10 years is characterized by exceptional liveliness in the research area as well as by pronounced shifts in research emphasis and in investigator role. Since space does not permit comprehensive coverage, only illustrative studies conducted and published in this country for 1965-1975 can be cited. One such sampling, representing a particularly active area,

Table 1. Perception research: illustrative studies 1965-1975		
Investigator and Research Topic	Test/Task and Deaf Sample	General Results
Visual Perception Gilbert & Levee (26) Visual-perception influence on test performance	Archimedes Spiral; Bender-Gestalt	Deaf significantly inferior on both tests
Doehring & Rosenstein (11) Speed of visual perception	Visual perception speed test 50 deaf, 10.9-14.9 years	Deaf inferior on 9 of 13 test items Older Ss superior to younger
Lawson & Myklebust (40) Visual defect incidence; relation to learning	Visual/opthalmological tests 80 deaf, 4-10 years	Deaf twice as many visual defects No direct relation to learning
Keogh, Vernon, & Smith (37) Visuo-motor skills; validity of Bender-Gestalt	Bender-Gestalt 160 deaf, 96-203 months	Deaf visuo-motor performance depressed ● Bender-Gestalt dubious for deaf children ● individual differential diagnosis
Sanders & Coscarelli (64) Relation between visual synthesis and lipreading	Utley Lipreading; Visual Closure; Disemvoweled Words; Missing consonant sentences. 24 deaf, 19-60 years.	Significant correlation between visual synthesis skills and lipreading
Color Perception Suchman (75) Color-form preference	Color-form discrimination; accuracy discrimination; discrimination learning tasks 36 deaf, 7.6-12.3 years	Most deaf Ss prefer color Most hearing Ss prefer form
Frey & Krause (16) Color perception	Dvorine PI Vision Test; Archer Word list 308 deaf, 9-18 years	Deficiency in deaf color-discrimination greater than twice that of general population
Tactile/Tactual Perception Schiff & Dytell (66) Tactual information processing	Battery of 7 tactile/tactual tests 179 deaf, 7½-9½ years	Deaf equal to or better than hearing on 6 of 7 tests
Blank & Bridger (5) Visual/tactile cross-modal transfer	Discriminate something/nothing; quantity discrimination 24 deaf, 2.11-5.4 years	Deaf more proficient than hearing in using tactile cues
Social Perception Michael & Kates (50) Social-concept attainment	32 2-person thematic cards: adult/child; day-/night-clothes; female/male; smiling/frowning 20 deaf, M. 201 months	No deaf-hearing differences in concept-attainment efficiency or strategies
Kates (33) Perception and interpretation of love/anger movement patterns	Filmed faceless rectangles in movement patterns for love and anger 32 deaf adults	No significant deaf-hearing differences in 'high anger,' 'high love,' 'medium love' movement interpretations ● Significant difference in deaf interpretation of 'medium anger' as 'high anger'
Schiff & Saxe (67) Judgment of personality traits from kinetic and facial information	Films of interactions of actual people and of real faces deaf college students	Marked deaf-hearing differences, with deaf giving more weight to body-motion information, and hearing to facial expression
Schiff (65) Social perceptions and interpretations	Four social perception tests incorporating visual cartoons and cartoon films 113 deaf, 12-19 years	Striking deaf-hearing differences in interpretation of hostile social interaction based on gross motor activity

is presented in Table form and includes selected studies related to cognitive processes. Studies in other categories are noted in the course of the discussion that follows which summarizes the shifts that have taken place in research direction and investigator role, and concludes with a summary-overview.

Cognition. Studies in the category of cognition occupy the major focus of activity in the past decade. Of the impressive total number, only a few could be accommodated in Table 2. Although still goal-oriented toward an investigation of mental functioning in a context of deafness, the studies have veered away from the old I.Q. approach, and, led by Furth, have centered instead on the processes involved in cognition and perception, and on Piaget theory testing (17, 19).

Table 2.   Cognitive processes: illustrative studies 1965-1975

Investigator and Research Topic	Test/Task and Deaf Sample	General Results
Conrad & Rush (8) Nature of imagery in short-term memory of 'verbal' material	Memorize 5-consonant sequences 41 deaf, 13-20 years	Deaf significantly poorer Nature of imagery undetermined
Youniss & Furth (88) Influence on discrimination of word meaning *vs* word appearance	Synonymous word-pairs; similarly appearing word-pairs 30 deaf, 12-15 years; 20 deaf college level	Younger deaf more influenced by word appearance Older deaf as influenced as hearing by word meaning
Lantz & Lenneberg (39) Influence of verbal reinforcement on short-term memory	Color perception-and-memory task 30 deaf, 6 years; 38 young adults	No deaf-hearing difference in perception Deaf children inferior in color memory No memory inferiority in deaf adults "Language increases amount of information a person can store" (p. 777).
Ross (62) Prediction of chance events	Two-choice probability tasks of varying uneven odds, even odds, and 'sure thing' outcomes 20 deaf, 11-15 years	Younger deaf two years behind hearing Older deaf "catch up" with hearing
Withrow (86) Effects on immediate recall of rate and method of stimulus presentation, meaningfulness, and number of items per trial	Silhouettes of: familiar objects; familiar geometric forms; random, geometric forms 52 school-age deaf	Deaf and hearing same in simultaneous presentation Hearing significantly superior in sequential presentation
Kates (34) Symbol-concept learning and reasoning	Decoding sentences composed of learned arbitrary symbols for 'and,' 'or,' 'not,' and alphabet symbols for color 16 deaf, 11-17 years	Deaf as able as hearing in learning and using symbols for logical concepts
Robertson & Youniss (61) Mental imagery in operational intelligence	To imagine water level in rotated bottle To imagine shadow-forms projected by rotated object 16 deaf, 98-117 months; 16 deaf, 135-155 months	Equivalent performance of deaf and hearing within Piagetian framework
Youniss, Furth & Ross (89) Symbol/concept learning and reasoning	Decoding and indicating true-false of sentences composed of learned arbitrary symbols for shape, color, negation, conjunction, inclusive-disjunction 48 deaf; 9.3-13.7 years	Deaf inferior in quantitative score and lag behind hearing in developmental pattern of learning and reasoning
Hoeman, Andrews & deRosa (31) Influence of sign-language reinforcement in short-term memory of deaf	Naming of previously presented pictures of common objects; color naming 31 deaf; 8-12 years	No difference in short-term memory encoding with deaf using sign-language reinforcement equivalent to verbal reinforcement used by hearing
Becker (4) Comparison of deaf and hearing cognitive strategies	Concept abstraction and matching for shape, color, number	Performance of deaf poorer at all age levels but same range of strategies characterize both deaf and hearing

The rationale behind the move is that, since the normal mental potentials of the deaf had long been established through decades of performance intelligence testing, no special purpose is served in belaboring the subject with continued I.Q. studies, particularly in view of their gross inadequacy in providing leads and insights to account for the poor showing of the deaf in learning-related accomplishments.

The new approach sought to provide new knowledge by digging beneath the surface of the I.Q. with Piaget test-tasks in order to get at some of the basic processes involved in deaf information processing, particularly in the cognitive area. The assumption was that the strategy would provide a more refined method for ascertaining if there were any malfunction within the deaf information-processing system itself, which, while not discernible in the I.Q., might nevertheless be present and so account for problems of the deaf in the acquisition and application of knowledge. If no inner malfunction were found, it could be reasonably assumed that the answer to deaf deficiencies must lie outside the deaf person in such learning-obstructing influences as experiential and linguistic deficits and communication handicaps.

While it is true that several studies along these lines have been previously attempted, the difference between them and the more recent ones is that the former were relatively isolated investigations, whereas the studies of Furth, his associates and followers, are linked together in a frame of Piaget theory which provides the investigator with a criterion-guide for evaluating results, and at the same time provides the theorist with a unique deaf population for theory testing.

These advantages are, however, cold comfort to uninitiated readers of both Piaget and Piaget-inspired investigations since the research reports tend to echo the master's abstruse, neologistic terminology, which requires its own special dictionary (3) as well as a legion of interpreters (15, 6, 55, 18) to cite only a few. Hence, it is safe to say that an evaluation of the studies in depth has escaped the critical eye of the field of the deaf and that the studies themselves have made less impact on the field than have the investigators' personal interpretations and extrapolations of their findings which are generally reported in ordinary language.

One of the paramount contributions to the 'new knowledge' advanced by these studies is that no basic malfunctions are present in the cognitive capacities of the deaf and that whatever inferiorities may be found in cognitive competence can be accounted for by experiential and linguistic deficits and communication handicaps. This is pretty much the way in which the old I.Q. investigators viewed the picture. What is more, it is derived in pretty much the same way, namely through a type of nonverbal performance testing. True, the Piaget tasks are highly ingenious and more mentally challenging. Nevertheless, they belong to the family of performance tasks. What is missing from the strategy as used with the deaf is Piaget's crucially important 'clinical interview' method whereby he was enabled to probe into the thinking and reasoning that governed the test performances of his subjects. Without this, all that shows is a subject's response. Thus, a hearing subject and a deaf subject may come up with the same response, but the cognitive paths that led to the respective solutions may be entirely different. Cognitive researchers have as yet failed to disclose the paths used by deaf subjects.

Another contribution of the Piaget investigators is that verbal language is not necessary for logical thinking. This too is scarcely 'new knowledge,' having been successfully demonstrated many millennia ago when prelinguistic man decided he needed a verbal code to help him up the ladder of civilization, and then proceeded to invent one—all without benefit of the word. That thinking is possible without verbal language is demonstrated in many other ways: in animal problem solving

(59); in the thinking and reasoning of prelinguistic babies; and in the many nonverbal thoughts that pass through the minds of us all in the course of a day in the form of concepts imbedded in feelings, creative imagery, memories, and other concepts. All these can be completely nonverbal before we coat them in words.

A final contradiction enters the cognitive research picture. When deaf subjects perform their Piaget tasks up to hearing standards, this is heralded as evidence that verbal language is not necessary to logical thinking. But when deaf subjects fail to reach hearing standards, language deficits are held as a responsible factor. This is a form of circuitous reasoning that is hard to follow.

What the cognitive studies seem to be saying is that deaf pupils possess the basic cognitive capacities for thinking and reasoning on a par with hearing peers, but that actual cognitive competence may be depressed to a greater or lesser degree as a result of linguistic, experiential, and communicative deficiencies. This is hardly new knowledge. The key inquiry that initiated cognitive research with the deaf remains unanswered, namely what is the nature of the cognitive processes and imagery that sustain thinking and reasoning in a context of deafness.

Intelligence and achievement. The shift in research emphasis from I.Q. to cognitive studies has by no means wiped out investigations of intelligence, but there is a shift in emphasis here too. Studies dealing mainly with psychometric issues and deaf-hearing I.Q. comparisons have taken a back seat to studies comparing deaf children of deaf parents with deaf children of hearing parents in intelligence and/or achievement.

Abridged digests illustrating the psychometric-type studies are as follows: the use of the Hiskey-Nebraska Test as a predictor of academic achievement, with equivocal results (25); investigation of the test-retest reliability of the Chicago Non-Verbal, the 1938 Raven's Matrices, and the Terman Non-Language Multi-Mental tests with a finding of significant increase in retest scores on all tests (29); construction of a new performance scale of cognitive capacity for the deaf consisting of such familiar test items as the Knox Cube, Alexander Passalong, Binet Beads adaptation, a Form Assembly task, and a Block Design task (36); a deaf-hearing group comparison using Raven's 1947 Colored Matrices that showed no significant difference between the groups (30); and a comparison between teachers' rankings of intelligence and the test results obtained from the Leiter International Performance Scale and the Raven's Colored Matrices, with the finding of no difference between teacher evaluations and test results for each scale (52). Of particular interest to the writer was a 1970 study (63) which harks back to one conducted by the writer some two decades ago in which the full Wechsler Adult Intelligence Scale was used for a comparison of verbal and performance I.Q.s. (42). The 1970 study found a 34-point difference between the two in favor of the Performance Scale and pointed out the sharper predictive value of the Verbal I.Q. in certain areas, as opposed to the Performance I.Q. The inferences of these findings warrant closer attention than has been accorded. To sum up, it is obvious that studies such as the foregoing are of interest mainly to the psychometrically concerned. They have created no great stir in the field of the deaf.

The stir-creating studies of the past decade are the deaf-deaf comparisons of intelligence and/or achievement. These are abridged as follows: comparison of the educational achievement of deaf children of deaf parents with that of deaf children of hearing parents (72); study of the influence of early manual communication on linguistic development (74); a comparison of deaf children of deaf parents with deaf children of hearing parents in intellectual, social, and communicative functioning (51); comparison of intelligence quotients of deaf children of deaf parents and those of deaf children of hearing parents (7); investigation of the influence of fingerspelling on language, communication, and educational achievements (57); comparison of the educational achievements of deaf children of deaf parents with those of deaf children of hearing parents (84); the effects on educational achievement of oral preschool education, early manual communication, and no preschool education, but with hearing parents (85); and a series of studies investigating the influence of early manual communication on achievement, communication, and adjustment (69). The overall picture obtained from these studies is one of general superiority of the deaf children exposed to early manual communication by reason of deaf parents. This obtains for most areas of inquiry, particularly for the key area of reading in which superiority is reported as statistically significant, as it also is in the Brill comparison of intelligence quotients.

In contrast to these findings are the studies in defense of oralism (38, 60). Lane compared the reading scores of 132 orally-educated former pupils of the Central Institute for the Deaf with the scores reported in the Wrightstone study (87), and in the Vernon and Koh (85) investigation, and found the reading scores of her oral sample exceeded those of the Wrightstone sample by 2.2 grades, and were comparable to the reading scores obtained by Vernon and Koh for their manual group. Rister reports that 81.9% of the 55 oral mainstream deaf children of her survey received "adequate achievement" ratings by their regular school personnel. Research evidence in defense of oralism over the past decade scarcely balances that promoting manualism in either amount or clout.

The sharp shift in the focus of I.Q. and achievement research to comparisons of children from orally favored vs manually favored backgrounds has had a strong impact not only on the field but also on related research, with increasing numbers of reports taking manual positions. However, what the findings per se actually reveal is that the superiority of the manually reared children in terms of absolute amounts is generally not as great as the designation "statistically significant difference" would suggest. As Quigley (57) points out in regard to several such studies (74, 51, 57), the differences obtained "were not large even when statistically significant" (p. 94). In reading, they rarely exceeded one grade. Similarly, in the previously cited Brill study (7), the difference of 9 I.Q. points in favor of the manual group, while statistically significant, has no practical significance in either psychometric theory or practice. Nonetheless, the smallness of the differences has not dampened the ardour of the investigators, which certain analyses indicate is considerably stronger than the related research (54, 53).

Personality. Personality research with the deaf has suffered a sharp decline over the past decade. It may be that researchers are admitting defeat in their efforts to find a personality test that lends itself to traditional experimental design while at the same time doing justice to deaf subjects. Or it may be that researchers have come to accept the picture of the deaf that has emerged from decades of personality testing as one characterized by such traits as rigidity, immaturity, deficient adaptability, and various other traits suggestive of "maladjustment."

Over the past decade, findings along these "maladjustive" lines have emerged from studies using the Structured Objective Rorschach Test (SORT) (28); the California Test of Personality (78); and the Id, Ego, Superego Test (90). Possibly the most disturbing finding, and one that warrants question, is that derived from a mental health survey in which almost five times as many deaf as hearing pupils were reported to be severely emotionally disturbed (69). On the other hand, 160 deaf subjects obtained scores associated with normal adjustment on the Missouri Children's Picture Series (77). This is one of the rare personality studies in which such "normal" findings were obtained.

Finally, one personality study of the past decade sought to break away from "the" personality of "the" deaf approach by taking cognizance of the marked heterogeneity and sharp differences that characterize the deaf population (49). Using the Hand Test with three groups of deaf young-adult subjects that diverged widely *only* in respect to linguistic level and academic achievement, the investigators found the personality patterns were also widely divergent from group to group, with 20 out of 24 Hand Test variables significantly discriminating among the groups. This study marks a pioneer effort in personality research to give more than lipservice to the heterogeneity of the deaf population through relevent planning in research design and selection of subjects.

Investigator Role

Together with the shift in research emphasis, there has occurred a shift in the investigator role, with researchers of the past decade becoming active participants in implementing the findings of their studies. This is in direct contrast to the conventional stereotype of experimental investigator as one whose task is completed with the discovery of new knowledge. As Garner (23) caricatures the basic researcher, "the less contact the scientist has with the problems of the problem-solver, the more apt he will be to fill the public domain with knowledge of ultimately greatest import to the problem-solver" (p. 942).

It has not worked out this way in psychological research with the deaf. For one, most, if not all, the leading investigators have themselves worked closely with the deaf at one time or another as "problem-solvers" and are deeply familiar with this side of the picture. For another, most, if not all, have been driven to research out of deep frustration with the unchanging status of the deaf over the decades, and with the futility of expecting traditional educational measures to improve the situation.

Propelled by this double motivation, investigators have not hesitated to use their research as an advocacy weapon against the particular practices they considered responsible for the deficiencies of the deaf. Nor have they hesitated to use their research findings where supportive, or their interpretations and extrapolations where findings were equivocal, to actually initiate educational change.

For example, one investigator, having drawn conclusions from his research of the need of deaf children for practice in thinking and reasoning, has himself followed through with a book of "thinking games" based on Piaget tasks and theory (22). The games are now being utilized in various schools for the deaf. All the investigators cited in connection with the deaf manual-background *vs* deaf oral-background studies have actively participated in initiating educational change in line with their positions. Finally, a number of investigators, Furth and Vernon in particular, have disseminated their research findings, positions, and impact throughout a vast selection of professional journals representing a wide variety of disciplines.

To sum up, psychological researchers with the deaf have emerged from their traditional shells of quiet objectivity over the past decade and have become active participants in effecting change. This is an unprecedented role. Through their actions, increasing numbers of educators are harking at last to the recommendations of psychologists, hopefully for the best.

Overview

Whether the shifts in research direction and investigator role are matched by sharpened psychological perceptions of the deaf person remains to be examined. Piecing together the jigsaw of findings obtained from the various illustrative studies here mentioned, the emerging picture of the deaf school-age, adolescent residential-school pupil used in the majority of cited studies is somewhat as follows:

The individual is likely to have some type of visual defect that appears to have no direct effect on learning activities (40). Further, visual perception is apt to be inferior (26, 11), and visuo-motor skills depressed (37), while lipreading abilities depend to a considerable extent on the individual's visual synthetic skills (64). There is also apt to be a greater or lesser degree of color blindness present (16); yet the individual's personal preference is likely to be color rather than form (75). However, tactual/tactile superiority would be expected when compared with hearing peers (5, 66).

In the area of social perception, although no differences would be expected between our deaf individual and hearing peers in regard to efficiency or strategies used in social concept attainment (50), there ar e likely to be a number of differences in social perception, with the deaf individual relying more and sometimes mistakenly on social clues from body language and movement than from facial expression (33, 67, 65).

In cognitive capacity, no difference would be expected when compared with hearing peers, but in cognitive competence there is apt to be a greater or lesser degree of inferiority due to linguistic and experiential deficiencies and communication handicaps (Table 2).

If our research-assembled individual is the child of deaf parents, his/her superiorities over the deaf child of hearing parents are likely to be present in certain areas, with significant superiority expected in reading achievement and intelligence quotient (see page 30). Under certain circumstances, however, an oral background would appear to have no adverse effect on reading achievement (38, 60). In either case, reading achievement would be expected to be considerably inferior to hearing levels.

Finally, in the area of personality, such traits as rigidity, immaturity, and impulsivity may be present (28, 78, 90), and emotional disturbance would not be surprising (69).

To sum up, the composite picture here assembled shows no dramatic difference from that produced by investigations of previous decades. To those familiar with deaf children and adolescents, it is a singularly lifeless picture in which the individual's inherent temperament and assets are either entirely missing or else are buried under a pall of negative findings. But this is the expected outcome when an individual is pieced together from tests emphasizing simple, readily quantifiable responses, and from test findings of investigators following a single line of inquiry rather than joined in programmatic effort. In this connection, an illustrative comment seems appropriate. In calling attention to the "transactional" integrity of affect and cognition in the mapping of cultural space, Stevens (71) points out that "....by themselves, affective measures provide little information about the cognitive structures in which they are imbedded and cognitive measures provide little information about the affective structures that give them meaning....Without information about both affective and cognitive components of human-environmental behavior, one cannot adequately consider "learner characteristics"...which existentially involve the two" (p. 440, 441).

Chiefly responsible for the "sameness" of the psychological research picture of the deaf individual from decade to decade is the basic sameness of the instruments used. Not only is their appropriateness questionable in regard to deaf subjects, it is questioned in regard to all subjects. As Cronbach (10) views today's tests:

   . . . my overall impression of today's practical tests . . . is that they are obsolescent. Tests that saw the light of day before 1949, with new norms and new scoring procedures, are in many areas the best we have today. . . . I cannot escape the feeling that the things actuarially scored tests cannot do are more important than the things they can do. Is the time not ripe for a wholly fresh effort to construct a new generation of tests? (p.xxvii).

Needless to say the time is more than ripe for new approaches in psychological research with the deaf. One that might be pursued—and this with the basic intent of deriving information rather than scores—is the development of "situational tests" (1, pp. 605-612) in which the individual is placed in a simulated real-life type of situation somewhat similar to the worksample technique used vocationally, excepting that the target of inquiry would be personality variables. As for the real-life test situations themselves, there should be no great difficulty in assembling a pool derived from and suited to the life situations of deaf persons. Further, to simplify the procedure, cinepsychometric techniques (70) might be used so that the real-life situation could be presented in film form. Granted, such a project would require multidisciplinary talent and team effort of no mean order as well as long term investment and funding, but it would be well worth the time and effort to escape from the test-cage in which psychological research with the deaf has been entrapped for so long and with such modest returns. A current approximation to this approach can be found in the social perception studies in Table 1. Investigations in this relatively unexplored area (68) should be vigorously pursued.

Other investigations of value might include studies of the degree of equivalence in connotative meaning among messages similar in basic content but presented to a variety of selected subjects through different modes and situations of communication, i.e. oral, verbal (print), sign language, fingerspelling, total communication; person to person, lecturer to audience, via film. Also, the findings of various perception studies warrant follow-up investigation, as, for example, the possible presence and effects of color blindness on a deaf subject's performance on such colored psychological tests as Raven's Colored Progressive Matrices and the Rorschach Test; and the implications of visual deficiencies among the deaf for the uncontrolled use of visual instructional media and materials in the classroom. Research also needs to be directed to follow-up evaluations of the outcomes, successes, and failures of the various types of psychotherapeutic interventions presently being used with the deaf in the treatment of the emotionally disturbed, multihandicapped, psychotic, addictions, and the like. And, of course, the as yet unresolved question of instructional communication methods and language outcomes continues to call for finely designed and controlled long-term study. In this connection, Kates (35) has conducted a particularly well conceived series of studies comparing the language development of deaf adolescents trained by different methods, while Quigley (58) enters the psycholinguistic domain with a five-year investigation of the syntactic patterns governing the "grammar" of the deaf.

In view of the great pressure of unmet research needs in the field of the deaf, it is somewhat disconcerting to find that "hearing impairment was the only handicap in respect of which more grants were made for demonstration projects than for research projects" by USOE for the period 1964-1969 (32, p. 194). It may be that the funding of individual grants will have to give way to the funding of sustained interlocking research centers with stable rather than "migrant" personnel who are not under the anxieties of grant-renewal, the pressures of grant and report writing, the need to publish or perish, but who are granted the right of scientists to move with courage, vision, new approaches, inventive techniques into the "big-problem" research posed by that unique "experiment in nature" (42, p. 11), the deaf population. The deaf deserve no less.

5

Glenn T. Lloyd, Ed.D. and
Douglas Watson, Ph.D.

Social and Rehabilitation Services:
An Emerging Force in Deafness

Dr. Lloyd is associate director and Dr. Watson is director of service research at New York University Deafness Research and Training Center, New York City.

Social and rehabilitation services provided through state-federal vocational rehabilitation programs historically have comprised the primary service-delivery system for deaf adults in the United States. Whether providing direct-client case services on the local level, sponsoring regional evaluation and training centers or national vocational-technical training programs, vocational rehabilitation has invested considerable effort and funding into improving delivery of services to deaf adults (6).

It is only within the past decade (1965-1975), however, that these efforts have changed from isolated and uncoordinated duplications to a system featuring linkage and coordination, program planning, development, and evaluation on a national level. These developments have significantly enhanced the delivery of social and rehabilitation services to deaf adults. Large gaps remain, however, indicating the need to review and critically assess major program developments in planning for the immediate future. For deafness rehabilitation to maintain its progress toward achieving professional maturity and self-actualization as a field, we must reassess where we came from in order to better plan and coordinate the continued emergence of social and rehabilitation services as a viable force.

Program Planning and Development

The basic justification for social and rehabilitation service programs provided for deaf persons is that they provide a significant contribution for meeting the needs of these individuals and enhancing the quality of their lives. The acceptance of this assumption is readily apparent in the field of deafness rehabilitation. Practice and research in this field have placed a strong emphasis on utilization of population

34

studies to determine population size, characteristics, and associated service needs as the basis from which to derive program planning and development priorities (43). Program planning and development derived from population surveys and demonstration research projects sponsored by the Rehabilitation Services Administration (RSA) have played a significant role in improving delivery of services to deaf persons in several important areas.

Population Studies. The thrust of this strategy has evolved around the dimensions of population distribution, characteristics, and service needs that were derived from national, regional, and local population surveys. The unprecedented wealth of demographic and service priority information generated by studies (24, 36, 29, 3, 20, 10, 11, 34) during the 1960's laid the groundwork that stimulated program planning and development at all levels of the rehabilitation service delivery system. It was not until 1974, however, that the National Census of the Deaf Population (37) provided the kind of comprehensive and reliable population data the field requires.

The relative significance and impact of population survey research lies in the body of information and knowledge it generated about deaf persons and their service needs. By permitting a high degree of confidence on the part of program planners and funding agencies, population studies have contributed significantly to virtually every major program developed in deafness rehabilitation during the last decade.

Program planning and development, however, are directly determined by the quality and relevance of the information available to program planners. All of the studies cited above, although directly influencing program development efforts, comprised, at the best, only global estimates of population parameters. To maintain the momentum of the past decade and more productively employ its resources in the years ahead, the field needs to develop ongoing annual population studies to obtain reliable and updated planning information. An annual survey using the methodology and procedures developed by the national census (37) would be relatively inexpensive to maintain either on a state-by-state or national level. The model for a state-by-state inventory of rehabilitation services to deaf clients currently being developed by the Council of State Administrators of Vocational Rehabilitation (CSAVR) in conjunction with the New York University Deafness Research and Training Center (DR&TC) provides a viable mechanism to maintain an annual inventory of the characteristics and service needs of deaf clients at appropriate governmental levels (31). Annual surveys would circumvent the temporal constraints of prior population studies, where data are quickly out-of-date due to changing economic and population characteristics.

Services for Multiply Handicapped Deaf Persons. One of the early results of the population studies was the identification of a large segment of the deaf population with multiple and severe handicaps who required specialized treatment programs. A large number of comprehensive rehabilitation evaluation and training programs for multiply handicapped deaf clients were developed throughout the country in response to this need. Programs, such as those in Arkansas (7, 32), Missouri (19), Ohio (18), Illinois (16), Massachussetts (22), New York (2), and Indiana (26), were sponsored by RSA to research and demonstrate the feasibility of serving multiply handicapped deaf clients within general-purpose rehabilitation facilities.

These efforts demonstrated conclusively that a significant proportion of the multiply handicapped deaf client population could be effectively "mainstreamed" into ongoing rehabilitation facility programs, provided appropriate support staff and service were incorporated into the programs. Further, significant new sources of information, knowledge, techniques, and instrumentation were generated to enhance and facilitate rehabilitation efforts with this population sub-group (28, 12, 42,

40, 19, 32, 16). As a result, many other state vocational rehabilitation agencies have planned and developed ongoing facility programs for their multiply handicapped deaf clients.

Numerous problems remain, however. The size and distribution of the population limits the extent to which these services can be available to many individuals. Few cities, or in some instances, states, have a large enough deaf population to support the quality of services required. In many parts of the country, this has led to the development of regional centers that have the capacity for serving multi-state areas (e.g., Crossroads in Indianapolis and Seattle Speech & Hearing Center), but have the disadvantage of removing the client from the community in which he must eventually function.

Effective and valid treatment methodologies and instrumentation for use with deaf clients have not been developed. Confronted with demands for immediate service to clients, the field has been forced to borrow extensively from practices used with general clients. Too often these "borrowed" techniques are not even valid with general client groups, let along the unique needs of multiply handicapped deaf persons. Current efforts to develop standards and guidelines for the vocational evaluation of deaf clients (46) promise assistance in improving this situation and in promoting more attention to this critical area.

A third major problem area is the lack of facility and professional staff certification standards. Current practices permit any facility program or rehabilitation worker to work with deaf clients, regardless of skills and quality of services. To ensure a minimum quality standard in these areas, certification standards must be developed and observed. The Professional Rehabilitation Workers with the Adult Deaf (PRWAD), in conjunction with NRA and CARF, would appear to be the logical organizations to address this issue and provide the leadership necessary to ensure quality services for deaf clients.

Postsecondary Training Programs. Program planning and development, for those deaf persons identified as needing postsecondary vocational-technical training, have resulted in the establishment of more than 40 programs in community and four-year colleges throughout the country (30).

The establishment of the National Technical Institute for the Deaf (NTID), in 1966, provided the initial thrust in providing viable college-level alternatives for deaf students (15). The "triangle colleges" that followed (8, 25, 47), have promoted a large number of postsecondary facilities that have "mainstreamed" deaf students into their existing programs. Most of these postsecondary programs have accommodated deaf students by providing interpreting, notetaking, tutorial, remedial, counseling, and associated special support services.

Benefits available to deaf students are immediately apparent in terms of career and program alternatives, reduced expenses and travel, scope and quality of instruction, and social integration with hearing peers at an earlier point in career preparation. The growing number of deaf students who exercise the option for enrollment in these programs indicates the relevance and desirability of this approach to postsecondary training.

However, a number of questions related to postsecondary programs such as certification standards, duplication of programs, and actual student benefits remain to be addressed by the field. Administrators of postsecondary programs should consider commissioning program evaluation addressed to these questions. We suggest that assistance for these efforts may be arranged through PRWAD in conjunction with the Conference of Executives of American Schools for the Deaf (CEASD), the Council of American Instructors of the Deaf (CAID), and a qualified program evaluation team from an independent university. Such efforts could assist materially in the development and maintenance of minimum program standards for the postsecondary education of deaf students.

Model State Plan for the Vocational Rehabilitation of Deaf Persons. Sustained concern with and action in the planning and organization of statewide vocational rehabilitation services for deaf persons date from the 1967 Las Cruces, New Mexico meeting. Numerous "spin off" regional meetings followed, leading to the 1971 Tarrytown Conference (41), and culminating in the Model State Plan (MSP) (35).

The MSP, presenting comprehensive guidelines for program planning and development at the state level, comprises perhaps one of the most important products of the past decade. A product of coordinated efforts by CSAVR, PRWAD, the Deafness Research & Training Center, and a group of professionals from the state, regional, and federal levels, it already has helped to effect employment of State Coordinators for Services to Deaf Clients (SCD) in more than 40 states. MSP has also centralized statewide program planning, development, and coordination; and influenced the development of a PRWAD Section for SCD that promotes intercommunication for the sharing of ideas and problems. It has stimulated a current MSP inventory program involving CSAVR and the Deafness Research & Training Center, which will generate collection and analysis of client and program variables within each state upon which to base appropriate planning and program development. The MSP Inventory may provide a basis for regional and national planning where broader efforts are indicated.

Current assessment of MSP developments suggest that, though few states have implemented comprehensive state plans, substantial progress is underway. A major omission, perhaps, has been that the problems and needs of hearing impaired persons and those with other communicative disorders have not been addressed to date. A related problem is that deaf clients are viewed separately from other severely disabled client groups. The development and maintenance of an effective service-delivery system for deaf clients requires consolidation of funding, manpower, and facility resources, not segregation. Considering the current national economy and focus on centralization and consolidation of scarce resources, the field of deafness must inevitably come to grips with the need to expand its perspective and capitalize on existing and concurrent resources.

Mobilizing Community Resources. In actual practice, services for deaf persons have depended primarily on "mainstreaming" deaf clients into existing vocational rehabilitation evaluation and training centers, mental health treatment programs, postsecondary training programs, and associated resources available in the community. Philosophically, however, many leaders in the field still have not consciously accepted or recognized this service pattern; and, as a consequence, program development and maintenance are too often left to the discretion of decision-makers outside the field of deafness.

Research of service-delivery practice conclusively shows that the field needs to derive mechanisms for coordinated leadership of program planning and development. Further, these coordinated systems should be designed for maximum utilization of existing community resources in service to deaf clients (6, 14, 4, 5, 44).

Considering that the service needs of deaf persons extend far beyond the parameters of vocational rehabilitation and postsecondary training, it becomes obvious that the field must develop service-delivery systems that improve delivery of community-based services such as legal aid, housing, family planning, employment, and health-care, to deaf persons on an on-going basis (44).

The trend toward maximum utilization of community social service resources holds profound implications for social and rehabilitation service delivery to deaf persons. Traditional strategies of attaching deafness specialists to mental health or other community service programs, for example, are inadequate and often counterproductive. We need to change the functions of these limited manpower resources to those of program planning, development, and coordination which span the spectrum of all social service resources within the target community. Employing persons as program specialists, instead of in direct client services, promotes the development of an improved and expanded service delivery system that enhances and gradually increases the ability of general resources and service workers to serve deaf clients.

Beginning efforts in this direction are evident in the establishment of state commissions, such as those in Connecticut, Virginia, Utah, and Texas, which have responsibility for coordinating and monitoring state-wide program planning and development for services to deaf residents. Recent developments in the field (35, 44) further detail the mechanisms and procedures by which a small team of deafness program-specialists can plan, develop, and coordinate community-based systems for improving delivery of social services to deaf persons.

Still in the developmental stages, these service patterns offer implications for changes in manpower deployment, counselor preparation, funding, research, and improved service delivery, which need to be explored and debated in the field. The immediate and long-range consequences of these trends require our full attention and scrutiny should we desire to monitor and coordinate this emerging trend of service delivery.

Professional Training Programs

The development of professional training programs to prepare counselors and associated rehabilitation personnel for careers in deafness rehabilitation has significantly enhanced the quality and number of professionals thus engaged. In some instances, the training programs have been degree oriented, and in others, they have been short-term programs of three months or as little as one day. Regardless of duration and terminal skills, these programs illustrate the awakened consciousness at the federal level (RSA) of the need for preparation of rehabilitation personnel who possess the particular knowledge and skills necessary for effective delivery of services to deaf clients (48).

Graduate Training Programs. Seven major institutions distributed across the country, (New York University, Gallaudet College, University of Tennessee, Northern Illinois University, University of Arizona, California State University at Northridge, and the Oregon College of Education) have provided leadership over the past decade in the in-depth preparation of deafness rehabilitation specialists by offering specific disciplinary preparation for graduate degree candidates. Providing master's, specialist, and doctoral degrees, these programs further developed viable short-term training alternatives. Graduates of these programs have included a significant number of deaf professionals, many of whom have gone on to earn doctorates, mostly in rehabilitation fields. An increasing number (M.A. and Ph.D.) are being sought and appointed to even higher levels of administrative responsibility.

Many of the improvements in social and rehabilitation services for deaf persons must be credited, in great part, to the efforts of such programs as referred to here, and are certain justification for their continuation, support, and expansion. There remains, however, a number of modifications and/or the restructuring of training programs that needs to be considered and possibly incorporated by the field.

Although effective for preparation of counselors and administrative personnel, graduate training has neglected the need for preparation of other specialists in the numbers needed to bridge significant gaps existing in delivery of social services to deaf persons. This oversight suggests that we need to develop linkage with other speciality disciplines to mount conjoint training programs for preparation of professionals in priority service areas. Perhaps a feasible means of accomplishing this objective would be to integrate course work in deafness into existing graduate training programs in the helping professions to provide "preservice" training in deafness to general practitioners.

Practices in the field further indicate (44) the need for changes in the roles and functions of "deafness specialists" from direct services to those of program planning, development, and coordination. Training efforts need to remain abreast of these developments and provide the knowledge and skills required for preparation of "deafness program specialists."

Short-term Preservice and Inservice Training. The development of the graduate training programs listed above has made it increasingly possible to provide varying degrees of preservice and inservice training according to local conditions and needs. Personnel who deal with a deaf person only occasionally are able to obtain the type and depth of training best suited for their needs while others, with greater needs, may also be suitably served.

The University of Tennessee (3 months), Oregon College of Education (4 weeks), New York University (1-5 days), and Northern Illinois University (1-5 days) have Orientation to Deafness programs which are primary examples of short-term programs effective in increasing the knowledge and skills of general practitioners in service to deaf persons. More than 3,000 rehabilitation personnel, for example, have participated in the New York University Deafness Research & Training Center's Orientation program since 1973. More importantly, this program has been packaged (45), and is being utilized in other parts of the country without dependence upon outside personnel.

All the major training programs, supplemented by the National Association of the Deaf's Communicative Skills Program (NAD-CSP), provide ongoing training programs in manual communication. Consultant services, curriculum developments, texts, visual aids, and direct training are typical of program activities in communication skills training.

A more recent and, perhaps, more ambitious development in the communication area is the National Interpreter Training Consortium (NITC). In concept, this program is unique and holds promise for the future, as institutional, vested interests have been put aside in a common cause—to train interpreters across the nation. Programs (New York University, Gallaudet, University of Tennessee, St. Paul Technical-Vocational Institute, University of Arizona, and California State University at Northridge) participating in the NITC are utilizing their pooled resources to provide interpreter training in each state and region throughout the country (33). The potential of a consortium approach to training, as demonstrated by NITC, has far-reaching implications for training efforts in the field as a whole. We should consider, for example, the potential benefits of developing and maintaining closer coordination and cooperation in all major training efforts along the lines of the NITC, reducing duplication and competition for the purpose of rechanneling our resources to other need areas, such as psychology and vocational evaluation, which are currently not addressed.

Professional Organizations

Professional service organizations in deafness have provided advocacy and leadership underlying numerous major improvements and developments in social and rehabilitation service-delivery systems for deaf clients in the last decade. Providing a focal point and a forum generating ongoing dialogue, leadership, and coordination of effort, professional organizations have become a viable "third force" in the field. Organizational and interorganizational cooperative programing has promoted improved service delivery through several basic thrusts.

Organizational Development. At the beginning of the past decade, the only viable organizations in existence were those related to education, speech and hearing, and consumer groups. Professional and other groups concerned with social services for the adult deaf population generally lacked a viable forum through which to exchange dialogue and generate collective action. Recognizing the need for organizational leadership, concerned leaders in the field, in partnership with RSA, developed a number of major professional organizations that have played significant roles.

The Registry of Interpreters for the Deaf (RID), the first of several major organizational efforts on the national level, provided a vehicle for organization and certification of interpreters (39, 27). Shortly after RID was organized, the Professional Rehabilitation Workers with the Adult Deaf (PRWAD) was established as an interdisciplinary organization for professionals and others concerned with services to the adult deaf (21).

Expanding its traditional role and function as a primary social-cultural type of organization, the National Association of the Deaf (NAD) became a major influence. As the major consumer representative in the field, NAD assumed leadership in matters related to the delivery of professional services to the deaf community and worked in active partnership with allied professional, governmental, community organizations and institutions.

Two separate attempts to develop interorganizational coordination, the Council of Organizations Serving the Deaf (17) and Operation TRIPOD (13), met with initial success, but have not yet achieved their potential. Both these efforts appear to have been ahead of their time, and for the present maintain, at best, a dormant profile.

A significant consequence generated by these organizational efforts has been the development of close working partnerships with the National Rehabilitation Association (NRA) and its Council of State Administrators of Vocational Rehabilitation (CSAVR). These two organizations have become active and vigorous partners with the field of deafness, in its efforts to improve services for deaf persons.

Publications. A significant body of literature on deafness, for professional and lay consumption, has been generated during the decade by the NAD's publications office; PRWAD's *Journal of Rehabilitation of the Deaf, Deafness Annual,* and occasional monographs; RID; TRIPOD; COSD Annual Forums; and NRA's *Rehabilitation Literature.* Presenting a more accessible and current forum for information and knowledge exchange regarding developments in the field, the publication and dissemination of this literature has generated the mechanisms and platforms for professional education, growth, and leadership.

Organizational Programs. Conferences, conventions, and forums held by organizations in deafness have also proved invaluable for exchange of information and knowledge. A direct result has been more vigorous advocacy and leadership promoting increased awareness of program development priorities, which resulted in action by RSA and various states.

A prime example is NAD's National Census (37). The reliable deaf population data it provided is currently affecting RSA and state-level program planning and development efforts in service to deaf clients. The NAD, in conjunction with PRWAD and CSAVR, has further promoted and established a National Advisory Council to the RSA Commissioner's Office.

Another example is PRWAD - RSA, whose sponsored workshop for state coordinators for rehabilitation services for deaf clients (SCD) has promoted more and better exchange of ideas and cooperative efforts to improve services for deaf clients on the state-regional level (23). Conjoint efforts by PRWAD, NRA, CSAVR, and concerned leaders in the field resulted in the Model for a State Plan for Vocational Rehabilitation of Deaf Clients (35), which has had a profound impact on the field, generating unprecedented action and program development.

The NAD's Communication Skills Program, together with the National Interpreter Training Consortium (NITC) program for the training of interpreters and the RID's efforts in the area of interpreter certification, have promoted an increase in the quality and availability of professionals with manual communication and/or interpreting skills. This has directly influenced (increased) the capacity of existing community resources (colleges, mental health, rehabilitation, and associated programs) to "mainstream" deaf clients into their programs vis-a-viz utilization of staff with manual communication skills and/or interpreting support services.

Comprising an obviously effective "third force" in the field, these organizational efforts although productive are still in the developmental stages. We anticipate that, with the maturation and continued leadership of these organizations in the coming decade, the field will witness even more vigorous and productive developments in delivery of social and rehabilitation services to deaf persons.

Coordination and Consolidation of Programs. Although formal attempts to develop interorganizational organizations (e.g., COSD, TRIPOD) failed to achieve their potential, the numerous cooperative programs between various organizations (e.g., NRA, CSAVR, PRWAD, NYU, RID, NAD) have produced some of the more productive and significant program developments in deafness during the decade.

Developments during the last few years suggest that major organizations recognize that continued leadership and developments require consolidation of organizational memberships and programs into a more unified front. For example, NAD, in an "Open Letter" (38) has strongly urged two major service organizations to unite into a single organization in order to improve their operational effectiveness. The proposed unification, it was posited, would enhance their position with the deaf community, and provide a focal organization for improved communication and interaction with other organizations and governmental agencies.

Conclusion

Overall, the developments briefly discussed are significant in that they represent a giant step toward improvement of program planning and development, increased availability of services, and increasing interorganizational and interagency cooperation. Although a number of experimental programs have not become self-sustaining, the specialized needs of deaf people have been recognized as valid and worthy of meaningful, coordinated action by concerned individuals, organizations, and institutions. It appears that the decade now beginning will allow greater consideration and concentration on meeting the needs of deaf people and an ever-widening array of social services will be realized. We must not, however, merely assume that these improvements will occur. We must move together as individuals, as programs with common goals and cooperative efforts, and as consolidated-cooperative organizations to bring these goals to fruition.   ⚗

6

George W. Fellendorf, Ed.D.

International Trends

Dr. Fellendorf is executive director of the Alexander Graham Bell Association for the Deaf, Washington, D.C.

International exchanges take their most direct form when they are made in person, and during the period from 1966 to 1976 a number of world congresses made personal contacts possible. One group of international meetings on deafness was sponsored by the permanent World Federation of the Deaf (WFD) with headquarters in Italy. Another group of meetings was sponsored by what might be loosely called the "international congresses committee," a euphemism for a group of national leaders which has assumed responsibility for accepting the invitations of various countries for international congresses on education of the deaf.

International Meetings

Those meetings sponsored by WFD were organized largely around the psychological and social problems of hearing impaired persons of the member countries. A well organized set of permanent commissions of WFD provides some continuity to the topical areas of concern, a feature not found in the international congresses on education of the deaf. In essence, the WFD congresses have served to give hearing impaired leaders an opportunity to demonstrate their ability to organize and manage large international congresses. Professional educators have been conspicuously scarce at these meetings. This recognition has not been lost on the hearing impaired leaders striving to be regarded as equals by the professionals who traditionally have held the responsibility for their education. Perhaps because of this concern to be recognized by the professionals, and sometimes expressing itself in a form termed "deaf power," the hearing impaired leaders have found their international meetings primarily attractive to hearing impaired persons and to those professionals from developing nations who find a place on the program an appropriate reason for sponsored travel abroad. A frequently heard criticism of the Congress of the World Federation of the Deaf (1975), in Washington, D.C., was that the professionals from the United States did not support it through submitted papers or their presence.

On the other hand, the international congresses on education of the deaf held in Stockholm (1970) and in Tokyo (1975), in addition to the international conferences on oral education in Northampton and New York (1967), tended to attract more professional educators and clinicians than hearing impaired persons. Thus, there has been a tendency for the professionals to support those congresses in which the educational and clinical aspects, rather than the sociologic and psychologic aspects, of deafness are given higher priority.

Personal Travel and Exchanges

Winston Churchill Scholarships made it possible for a number of educators from Australia to travel to the United States and Europe for learning and exchange. Professionals from universities and associations in the United States have obtained sabbatical leaves for international visits that have stimulated personal and professional exchange. The foreign lecturer series of the A.G. Bell Association for the Deaf has brought to the U.S. such outstanding authorities as Dennis Fry (U.K.), Armin Löwe (GDR), Pierre Gorman (U.K.), Darcy Dale (U.K.), and Anthony van Uden (Netherlands). Through this innovative program, each has had the opportunity to deliver lectures and to receive information from colleagues in the United States. In addition, there have been actual exchanges of posts, such as that between Lutheran pastors for the deaf Daniel Porkorny of the United States and Edward Kolb of Switzerland, in which each assumed the pastorate of the other for a year.

Of utmost significance to the education of the hearing impaired in the United States was the visit of Boris Morkovin to the USSR in the early 1960's, whereupon he returned with reports dealing with successful use of fingerspelling with very young Russian hearing impaired children (1). Morkovin's knowledge of the Russian language added a great deal of authenticity to his reports of 2,000-word vocabularies mastered by the Russian children, as compared to 50 words of American children of the same age and hearing loss.

UNESCO, as the arm of the United Nations concerned with children in developing countries, convened a group of 13 experts who met for a week in Paris in October, 1974. Their shared experiences resulted in recommendations on education of the deaf for UNESCO consideration (2). In general, the experts emphasized the teaching of speech to deaf children as the more desirable communication mode for integration into the society of a nation. Selection of deafness as the first area to be investigated in this new UNESCO thrust was based upon the feeling that it represented one of the most difficult of the handicaps to manage. The meeting format proved successful and will be used as a model for UNESCO conferences concerned with other handicapping conditions.

Export and Import of Techniques

During the past decade some specific techniques have been exported from nation to nation, often on the basis of undocumented claims and frequently with an unusual amount of public relations. The *verbotonal* procedures of Petar Guberina of Zagreb, Yugoslavia, arrived in the United States and other nations in the mid-1960's and stimulated renewed interest in methods of using the residual hearing of even severely deafened children. *Acupuncture*, an ancient Chinese procedure for anesthesia, following President Nixon's historic visit to the People's Republic of China in 1972, suddenly appeared on the scene as the way to "cure" nerve deafness. Political, as well as medical, uneasiness accompanied the establishment of clinics in the United States to apply acupuncture to "cure" hearing impaired children and adults. However, failure to document a single case of cured nerve deafness eventually resulted in closing the clinics and ending their founders' dreams of fortunes. *Cued speech*, on the other hand, was exported from the United States to Australia, to the United Kingdom, and to other nations. It has found acceptance among those who have sought a way of improving speech skills using cues with speech rather than using silent signs. *Total communication*, still largely unsubstantiated for marked improvements in speech and language of all hearing impaired children, has passed rapidly from the United States to other nations. Often the transfer has been more on the basis of hearsay rather than any bona fide research by authorities of any of the nations involved. Although the term originated in the United States, the technique of using fingerspelling, signs, and speech simultaneously has been present for many years in most nations of the world. Countries that have traditionally been totally oral in their educational programs and philosophy have begun experimenting, and in some instances have converted freely to total communication methodology.

Evaluation of Events

The role of the United States as a leader in the area of the education of the hearing impaired appears to be well established although colleagues in many nations express doubts about some of the procedures adopted in the U.S.A. and exported elsewhere. An undue portion of U.S. leadership may be based upon the relative availability of funds for research and demonstration, and upon funds to publish, and to travel for the purpose of publicizing the results of studies. The most commonly accepted area of United States' leadership is probably in the area of secondary and postsecondary educational programs. A common expression heard from non-U.S. residents is, "Of course, only the United States has a Gallaudet College." Now, with the National Technical Institute for the Deaf, there is even further basis for claiming leadership in the higher education area. One must acknowledge, however, that in many other nations, entry to institutions of higher education is reserved for only the superior students, and frequently requires at least two foreign languages in addition to the mother tongue. Thus, higher education is more accessible in the United States for all students, including those with educationally handicapping conditions. It is likely that other nations will eventually try to replicate this model, at least in the case of the severely hearing impaired at the higher education level. In the meantime, talented foreign deaf students, who have a command of English, will try to enroll at Gallaudet, NTID, or one of the other programs having special facilities for meeting the needs of the deaf student.

International conferences, while continuing to provide opportunities for professional exchanges, are fast becoming prohibitively expensive. It is currently difficult to travel abroad under federal grants, and the advantages of such travel are difficult to justify. It appears that the day of large international conferences in the area of hearing impairment may be on the wane.

The expression "familiarity breeds contempt" suggests the tendency to look abroad for new ideas to meet the problems faced at home. *Cued speech* has been received more enthusiastically and has more retention in Australia and in the United Kingdom than in the United States where it originated. For a time at least, the *verbotonal* method was adopted widely in Belgium; while in Yugoslavia, where Guberina still practices, it is only one of the procedures used. The one exception to this phenomenon of familiarity may be *total communication*.

In the United States, it has always been possible to find a combination of fingerspelling and signs along with some speech, particularly with older deaf children. It was the rare oral school that could successfully maintain a strictly oral environment in the playground as well as in the classroom, particularly after the students reached adolescence. Thus, when total communication surfaced as a "new" method, many educators refused to acknowledge it as anything but the old combined system. As an acceptable method of instruction, and as a philosophy, however, it was rapidly accepted in many schools, clinics, and teacher preparation centers. Its future was enhanced in this country when the U.S. Bureau of Education for the Handicapped, which funds many special education research and demonstration programs, adopted the philosophy that deaf children should be offered forms of instruction that had at any time seemed to work for at least some children, some of the time.

Thus the term "total communication" arrived and was accepted by many in the U.S.A. At the same time missionaries, both personal and in the media, took off for the foreign shores and found a ready audience for what was billed as the new technique that had already taken over America. What was not always shared with foreign colleagues was that many educators and adult deaf persons in the U.S.A. were yet to be convinced that the educational needs of deaf persons, and especially children with severe to profound hearing losses, were being met by total communication as practiced in the United States.

In fairness to the total communication movement, it should be stated that its success both in the United States and its ready acceptance in a growing number of foreign countries is a reflection of the feelings of frustration that have plagued so many conscientious teachers and parents who have tried the totally oral way with all hearing impaired children. For a variety of reasons, many of which were not the fault of the child, usable auditory/oral communication did not result. With this as a background, it is understandable why the total communication philosophy was accepted by so many in the United States and elsewhere.

Integration of hearing impaired children into regular schools and classes has been practiced in the United States, the United Kingdom, and in Sweden over the past decade. This approach has had the desirable effect of forcing educators and policy makers to differentiate between partially and profoundly deaf students. This in turn has required many to review their use of terms and their historical positions regarding which children should be educated in which environment. However, optimism has sometimes overpowered good sense, resulting in failure of some children to achieve as expected because of improper, untimely placement, a lack of prepared teachers, and sometimes due to the insensitivity of administrators. In many nations, there were youth who were given the chance to mainstream but were not followed up with proper support. For this reason, and because of other school problems of finance and training, most nations have continued the practice of educational placement of deaf children in residential settings, while sending those with adequate language and speech skills into some kind of integrated program.

The Future

As international travel becomes more expensive, personal exchanges in the form of conferences and meetings will probably be reduced. Unless one can coordinate a vacation abroad with a professional meeting, or unless the government of a nation is willing to finance attendance, there will be less and less travel as that which occurred in the 1960's. National budgets have tended to offer fewer, rather than more funds, for international meetings and conferences, so the chances for short-term foreign travel and professional exchanges will be lessened.

Longer-term exchanges such as sabbatical leaves and exchanges of positions with colleagues in other countries appear to be more beneficial and economical. Extended professional visits of 3 to 12 months, including exchanges of appointments where the language barriers have been overcome, may become more customary. In many respects, these should be more beneficial since the time to get to know the customs, educational practices, and the politics of a nation will be available, and the tendency to overlook important aspects affecting the education of hearing impaired children and adults will be reduced.

Where will new leadership occur in the next decade? It seems that the United States will remain among those nations with the resources and the incentive to investigate new techniques and technological devices, areas which require relatively large investments of funds. The tendency toward gadgetry and easy solutions to the difficult problems of improving the language, speech, and social skills of the hearing impaired, however, will probably tend to characterize the work of many researchers in the United States, whose environments are dominated by the relatively bountiful availability of federal funds. Perhaps a reduction in the amounts of federal monies, available for research and demonstration studies of hearing impaired persons, will result in a greater discernment and attention to the quality of proposed investigations, thereby leading to greater advances in the conquest of the real fundamental problems of the deaf and hard of hearing.

Leadership may also evolve from the Orient, where the trend toward teaching English as a second language in Japan has placed a special focus on problems and techniques of second-language instruction of the normally hearing child as well as the hearing impaired child. With this orientation and the technology that is so evident in the products of Japan, the drive and work ethic of this nation may well father the newest advances of the future.

There are inherent dangers in some types of international exchanges, however, and these may continue in the future unless national professional groups stimulate cooperation to a greater and greater degree. For example, there must be greater understanding of terms and practices as used in various countries, since they are frequently used differently. Even the term *deaf* is misunderstood and misused within the United States; and when one studies its use in England, Sweden, Sri Lanka, and the USSR, it is evident that there are many definitions of this basic term that one would think was clear to any authority on education of the deaf throughout the world. If nations expect to benefit from the work of each other and to share their accomplishments with others, all must be prepared to learn the semantics of the field as they are understood internationally.

The provision of rehabilitiation and social services to hearing impaired persons in the United States and in many other democratic nations of the world may well be modeled in the future after the work in socialistic countries like the USSR and Poland. Other nations whose democratic policies include similar types of health and welfare programs, such as the United Kingdom, Sweden, Holland, and Denmark, may also become models of service delivery to hearing impaired persons in rehabilitation, social services, and similar areas. Whether or not these programs can be made fiscally sound over long periods of time, and in times likely to include periods of economic depression or inflation, remains to be seen.

7

Ralph L. Hoag, Ph.D. and
Roy M. Stelle, Ph.D.

Teachers of the Deaf:
Artisans to Professionals

Dr. Hoag, currently chairman of the Council on Education of the Deaf Committee on Professional Preparation and Certification, and superintendent of the Arizona State School for the Deaf and the Blind, Tucson, served as coordinator of programs for the deaf, U.S. Office of Education, responsible for administration of Public Law 87-276 (1962-1966).

Dr. Stelle, currently secretary of the Council on Education of the Deaf Committee on Professional Preparation and Certification, is retired superintendent of the New York School for the Deaf, White Plains.

During the 19th century, schools for the deaf prepared their teachers informally using in-service techniques. The first teachers and founders of new programs learned their skills in other schools. Preparation was an apprentice-type training much the same as that for tradesmen or artisans who were prepared for their work in special crafts.

As time went on, more formalized programs of profession preparation for teachers were held in schools for the deaf and led by master classroom teachers. The first of these emerged in 1889, at The Clarke School for the Deaf under the leadership of Dr. Carolyn A. Yale. Similar effors followed at Gallaudet College in 1891, at the North Carolina School for the Deaf in 1894, and at Central Institute for the Deaf in 1914. These were primarily school-based programs as contrasted with college or university-operated programs which were developed much later.

In 1924, after a decade of discussion to raise the standards of teachers of the deaf, a committee was appointed to outline a training course that would contain recommendations to be followed by all "normal" schools or other programs involved in the preparation of teachers of the deaf. This developed at a meeting of the Conference of Superintendents and Principals (CONFERENCE)* in St. Augustine, Florida. Membership on this committee represented the three major organizations of the profession at the time.

---

*The Conference of Superintendents and Principals of American Schools for the Deaf became the Conference of Executives of American Schools for the Deaf in October, 1930.

The report of this committee was presented and adopted at the 30th CONFER-ENCE meeting in Frederick, Maryland, in 1926, and is referred to in the record as the "Yale Outline." It is interesting to note that, even then, there were strong feelings and support for a two-year program for the preparation of teachers. In spite of this, a two-year program was later considered to be an impractical load to be added to the courses already required for teaching in public schools. Recogniz-ing that the programs in this field accepted students with a high school diploma, an effort was make to upgrade the quality of programs, by recommending that appli-cants should have at least two years of training in a "normal" school. However, no further action was taken beyond the recording and publication of the report.

Attention again was focused on the problem at the 14th meeting of the CON-FERENCE in Knoxville, Tennessee, in 1928. The outcome of this meeting was the appointment of a new committee directed to: "a) Find out what they (teacher preparation programs) are doing, how they are doing it, and to obtain copies of their respective courses of training; b) To determine their attitude toward the adop-tion of the Yale Outline as a minimum standard."

Certification for Professional Recognition

After three years of work, the special committee appointed in 1928 gave its report at a meeting of the CONFERENCE in Fairbault, Minnesota. It was reported that 21 programs were engaged in the preparation of teachers and were already complying or were willing to comply with the Yale Outline. The report suggested that there was no uniformity of method, no uniformity of purpose, and no unified standard. Each school, it appeared, conducted its program with total independence from what was going on elsewhere.

In the meantime, the American Association To Promote the Teaching of Speech to the Deaf (ASSOCIATION)* independently formulated and announced a plan for the certification of teachers under its own organizational authority. The certificates were to be issued through the offices of the Volta Bureau, in Washington, D.C.

The question of who should be given authority for the certification process was then discussed among members of respective organizations. It was held that since the CONFERENCE represented the employing members of the profession, the CONFERENCE should be the logical organization to have this responsibility for the entire profession. This proposal was approved at the 1930 meeting of the CON-FERENCE in Colorado Springs, Colorado, and a new committee was appointed to further develop this program.

At the 1931 meeting of the Convention of American Instructors of the Deaf (CONVENTION) in Winnipeg, Manitoba, a tentative set of standards for the certifi-cation of teachers was presented to the CONFERENCE for consideration and adop-tion. The Executive Committee of the CONFERENCE asked the existing Committee on Certification of Teachers to draw up a plan based on the one that had been proposed by the CONVENTION. The final set of standards was later adopted and used as the basis for granting certificates to teachers.

The requirements included three levels of certification. These were identified as A, B, or C, each relating to the level of preservice education: baccalaureate, normal school, or high school. A one-year program of preparation to teach the deaf, fol-lowed by three years of successful teaching experience, was required for each level

---

*The American Association To Promote the Teaching of Speech to the Deaf was known later as The Volta Speech Association for the Deaf. It became the Alexander Graham Bell Associa-tion for the Deaf in June, 1953.

of certification. Special provisions were made for granting certificates to persons with more than 10 years of experience prior to the adoption of this program in 1931. Initially, all applications for certificates were handled by the editor of the *American Annals of the Deaf*. The CONFERENCE committee on certification also had been given responsibility for the review and evaluation of programs. This provided the basis for giving recognition to "approved" programs. The results of the committee's work in 1932 were reported in the *American Annals of the Deaf* in the September issue of that year. At that time, 14 programs had been reviewed and all were granted the status of "approved" programs.

It should be noted that all of the centers for teacher preparation so recognized were school-based in-service training centers. Worthy of mention, also, is the fact that by September 1932, 250 applications had been processed for certification. This was virtually a landslide expression of interest and endorsement by teachers who were already working in the field.

The Move to Higher Education

In 1934 New York University on the East Coast, through the efforts of the principal of the Lexington School, and San Francisco State College on the West Coast, in conjunction with the California School for the Deaf at Berkeley, announced programs for preparing teachers of the deaf. These were the first programs since the establishment of the program at Gallaudet College to be affiliated with accredited institutions of higher education.

Continuity of Committee Leadership

The success of such an important program depended a great deal upon the people appointed to the committee, and especially those who served in the roles of chairman and secretary. These persons were continuously responsive to input from members of all organizations interested in the education of deaf children.

First Standards Revision

In 1951, after two years of work, the secretary of the Committee on Teacher Training and Certification, proposed a revised set of standards for adoption by the CONFERENCE. This was an attempt to standardize programs and identify curriculum content that should be covered in course work offered in various teacher preparation programs. A minimum level of 26 college course-hours was proposed as the foundation for a program. The proposal, approved by the CONFERENCE at its meeting in Missouri in 1951, recognized the need for periodic reevaluation of programs and included a plan for accomplishing this as well. These standards remained in effect from June, 1951, to January 15, 1974. The responsibility for the operation of this program by the CONFERENCE ended in 1969.

Professionalization of Teachers

The most dramatic series of changes in schools took place after World War II. The changes were caused by rapidly advancing technology, recognition of the need for early education, steadily lowering entry-age for children into educational programs, the population explosion, and the increasing numbers of children with multiple handicaps. These changes complicated programming for deaf children and forced serious examination of existing practices and teaching techniques.

Population mobility, increased numbers of new programs, the information boom, new technology in amplification, and the effects of linguistic research on earlier concepts and techniques used for language development all created problems for those engaged in the preparation of teachers. The need for specialization in the profession was rapidly becoming apparent.

The turbulent 1950's ushered in the critical need for teachers as the numbers of programs increased rapidly. This developing crisis brought together the extensive forces that existed in the profession. Through the newly established coalition of organizations in the field, the Council on Education of the Deaf (COUNCIL), administrators, parents, and teacher educators worked cooperatively to gain the attention of the United States Congress regarding this problem. Their efforts resulted in the passage of Public Law 87-276 in 1958, which authorized the establishment of a scholarship-student aid program that, in turn, aided the expansion and strengthening of existing programs, as well as encouraging the development of many new programs.

Early competition for funding created many problems that required immediate attention on the part of leaders in the field. Credit for bringing order to the program should be given to those in leadership roles at the time. The advisory group brought together by the governmental agency administering the program, as required in the legislation, was responsible for shaping its future. As a result, many of the more urgent needs of the time were recognized and satisfied.

The Transition Period

The certification program initiated by the CONFERENCE provided recognition to teachers who completed the recommended minimum program for the professional preparation of teachers and by 1969, the last year that the CONFERENCE administered this program, over 5,600 qualified persons had applied for and were granted certificates. Since 1969 more than 5,800 additional certificates have been granted. The original 1931 standards, recognized and generally accepted, and the revised 1951 standards were used extensively as guidelines for the development of teacher preparation programs, standards for licensing teachers by states, teacher qualifications in state and local programs, and by the U. S. Office of Education for awarding of grants to institutions of higher education.

A number of national conferences were held during the years following the passage of Public Law 87-276. The first among these was the Virginia Beach Conference on the Preparation of Teachers, held in 1964. Others that followed included the series of conferences on professional standards by the Council for Exceptional Children (1965-1966), and the Colorado Conference on the Education of the Deaf (1967). All of these focused considerable attention on the problems of teacher preparation. The efforts of those involved contributed greatly to changes in programs that followed.

If one were to identify a single major influence for change in the 1960's, it would be the Virginia Beach Conference. This was the first time in the history of the education of hearing impaired persons that a meeting was held that involved representatives of virtually all the diversified interests in the field. The topic was the preparation of teachers. Participants, with their varied experiences, backgrounds, interests, and expertise, focused on a common problem.

One of the recommendations from this conference which, in a sense, was treated as a directive, stimulated action by each of the organizations of the COUNCIL into reorganization patterns. The recommendation stated that "national standards should be established by a single organization, representative of all or most of the persons involved in the teaching of deaf children and in the administration of teacher preparation programs." It was further recommended that the COUNCIL and the CONFERENCE cooperate in establishing a committee within the COUN-CIL to develop new standards for the preparation of teachers. The Advisory Committee for Programs for the Deaf in the U.S. Office of Education was responsible for organizing the meeting in Virginia.

Events occurred within the member organizations of the COUNCIL for several years following the Virginia Beach Conference. The work of two ad hoc task forces appointed jointly by the CONFERENCE and the COUNCIL was going on during this period (1968 and 1969). The Connor-Stelle Task Force worked on preparation requirements and certification standards for academic teachers. The Castle-Wycks Task Force addressed itself to preparation of vocational and other related special subject area teaching personnel. In July of 1969 in Berkeley, California, a new committee on professional preparation and certification was established by the Executive Board of the COUNCIL, and members were appointed. This action was taken following resolutions from its three member organizations that such a committee be established. This committee was then charged with the responsibility for working with all interested persons (administrators, teachers, teacher educators, federal, state, and local officials; organizations; and the community of the deaf) toward the development of a set of updated standards. It was hoped that the committee would produce a universally acceptable set of standards that could be effectively used for the upgrading and improvement of programs eventually affecting personnel who work with hearing impaired children in schools in the United States.

Standards Set by the COUNCIL Committee

The COUNCIL Committee on Professional Preparation and Certification prepared a combined report, developed from recommendations of the two task forces, as a draft of proposed standards. This was widely circulated by the committee to state agency personnel, university program representatives, teachers, schools and classes for the hearing impaired, and to the leadership of national organizations of the deaf. The topic of standards revision was put on the agenda of conventions of several national organizations. Open discussion meetings were held at these conventions to get input from as many interested persons in the field as possible.

It took the COUNCIL committee two and one-half years to complete its assigned task. The results of these efforts became the basis for the published document of "Standards for the Certification of Teachers of the Hearing Impaired." The standards were formally adopted by the COUNCIL with the consent and approval of its member organizations on January 15, 1972. These standards, in this period of our history, represent the beginning of a series of activities that will undoubtedly have to be implemented by the committee. Some of this is already underway and in process. However, there is no question that the general acceptance of the new standards marks another milestone in the illustrious history of this very special field. Their eventual effectiveness will be determined by the extent to which they are used and adopted by all those in the profession.　　　　　　　　　　🜨

8

William N. Craig, Ph.D.

Curriculum:
Its Perspectives and Prospects

Dr. Craig is superintendent of the Western Pennsylvania School for the Deaf, Pittsburgh.

In the main, current curriculum activities in the area of deafness follow trends established in the broader fields of education. It is the adaptations, therefore—the modification and application of principles, processes, and content for groups of deaf students—that provide the really unique contribution from educators of these deaf children. Recognizing the instructional challenges imposed by the interruption of normal language, speech, and hearing development, the educator may reorganize the immediate instructional goals, and with this selection of immediate goals, many variations and adjustments to the curriculum must follow. The concepts of societal living, for example, may first need to be taught as a complex of social interaction, with deaf students in the class learning to play selected roles. The language structures, spoken phrases, attention to auditory cues, signs, and related activities become joined as a second signficant goal in this lesson; a goal the educator of the deaf is uniquely qualified to address.

The present discussion will not attempt to justify or reconstruct the broader curriculum approaches, which have been discussed in detail elsewhere (see Selected References, page 140); rather, it will focus on the application of some of these approaches in selected programs for deaf students. Specifically, attention will be focused on the following questions:

What is the appeal of a systematic approach to early education?

What has the "open classroom" concept meant to educators of deaf children?

How has the concept of "mainstreaming" or partial integration altered the curricular approaches in schools for the deaf?

What is happening to educational technology in the instructional process?

52

How are special-purpose projects being incorporated into the school curriculum? These topics cover a broad spectrum of instructional interest for educators of deaf children. They do not represent all of the possibilities for innovation or development, but they do represent areas of active concern and current implementation. In essence, these topics represent what educators are talking about this year and will probably continue to examine in the immediate future.

Early Education

Preschool and early primary-level instruction has always held special interest for educators of deaf children. Deaf children are likely to have few language concepts or skills prior to the time that specially prepared teachers or therapists see them. Therefore, it is necessary to apply principles, introduce materials, and organize instructional sequences without reliance on prior training. The educator fully expects that skills learned "correctly" during these early years will accelerate the instructional process and increase the probability that the deaf child will more closely resemble his hearing counterpart in the school system.

To illustrate the nature of recent curriculum change, two broadly based programs which have been developed during the past few years, may serve as useful references: Verbotonal instruction (2), based on the work of Petar Guberina; and the Peninsula Oral School system (6), developed from a curriculum framework originally proposed by Hilda Taba. Interestingly, the proponents of each approach caution that their systems are not easily mastered but, properly implemented, can provide significant results. Some highlights from these two instructional programs may point to a current trend.

The Verbotonal system was developed originally from a rhythm-based technique for teaching foreign languages. Principles developed from this effort were adapted to the instructional needs of deaf children and have subsequently been used in programs in the United States, France, Canada, the Netherlands, and Brazil. Essentially, the curriculum evolves around an activity-oriented, auditory approach to teaching language, speech, use of residual hearing, and, through this frame of reference, reading and writing skills. Rhythmic patterns of language instruction are incorporated in all of this instruction in much the same way as the original foreign language techniques were employed.

The major components of Verbotonal instruction include the use of body movements to establish speech patterns and auditory perception of these patterns. Emphasis is placed on acoustic memory for these patterns, thus games and "play" activities are designed to provide longer periods of attention to these patterns. Language instruction is built into these activities, which are always placed in a meaningful context or normal situation. The language presented permits the child to take the initiative in organizing the games or activities. Hearing aid equipment employs vibrators for tactile stimulation and broad frequency amplification, which can be adjusted for selected frequency contours. The responses of this equipment can be adjusted to the deaf person's optimum field of hearing. The components of Verbotonal instruction form an interrelated package which can produce some excellent results.

As a curricular innovation, the significant considerations in Verbotonal instruction are the flexibility the system provides, and the incorporation of special skill learning into the normal active play patterns of young deaf children. Rather than a presentation of a set vocabulary or a limited approach to each instructional component, it provides a single set of basic principles for an instructional package in which the specific content is free to vary with the situation.

Similarly, the Peninsula Oral School approach provides for the consistent application of a set of carefully organized principles to the instructional program. Of particular interest is the sequence of cognitive strategies or tasks, leading through concept formation, interpretation, inference, and generalization, and then to application of principles. Basically, mental skills are developed through a sequence of questions and answers, and the child is provided with language to specifically facilitate this process, e.g., "What's missing?" "How are _____alike/ different?" "What must I do?" (to make something work) "I need_____." "I want _____." "Why?" "Describe it." On a scale of classroom interaction analysis, this approach would show high frequency of communicative patterns between the teacher and student. According to Grammatico (6), the behavioral objectives for preschool include "the child's developing listening skills, watching, imitating, using language spontaneously, developing concepts, making comparisons, inferring, expressing feelings (his own and others'), thinking independently, and producing correct speech sounds." Not all of these objectives are included in one lesson or series of lessons, but they do provide the basis of the program, and all activities, including play, are specifically geared toward this cognitive-linguistic interaction.

Skipping over a number of components, the emphasis on posing questions deserves note. This is particularly true when the response may have several dimensions. A simple response to a question leads to a second, more probing question and a more expansive response. The child's answer to "What happened?" is not considered sufficient; he, or someone else in the class, must go on to answer "Why?" or "How do you feel about that?" The key element appears to be imbedded in the relationship of language and experience. Although the objectives of the curriculum are carefully planned, the child is not encouraged to memorize facts as much as he is led to using concepts, inferring, comparing, and developing a process of understanding his environment. Some of the basic concepts emphasized involve change, cooperation, similarity, interdependence, causality, and sequential order of events.

These selected preschool projects from Pennsylvania and California seem to offer possible directions for curriculum development during the next few years. In each case, they have evolved from a very specific concept of instruction. Each component of the plan is consistent with the stated instructional objective. Teachers are specifically taught to implement the total program including communication and cognitive skill development. The emphasis on coordination does not extend, however, to an incorporation of the child into a rote system of education, but rather, it assures that the instructional program is expansive and sensitive to the child's level of skill development. This instructional direction or management, when combined with a program that encourages alternatives, should provide an effective balance for testing other innovations in curricular design.

Open Classroom Organization

One instructional innovation during the last 10 years is the move toward a less structured system described as the open classroom. The merits of this approach have been debated in the larger arena of public education, and adaptations of open classroom instruction have become a part of the instructional planning for deaf children in some schools. Basically, learning through action is considered a key principle in helping deaf children internalize concepts and develop symbolic expression in this system.

Although open to modifications, there are central components of the approach that can readily be adapted for deaf students. Procedures which appear to be particularly useful include: a) use of experience-centered themes; b) inclusion of individualized alternatives in the learning centers; c) provision for both small group and individual presentations; d) use of games and role-playing situations; and e) writing of contracts, and record-keeping devices. These components change the classroom approach by encouraging the learner to choose from among a number of activities and to pursue them at a pace that he sets for himself. Classroom interaction analysis systems (3) applied to the open classroom for deaf students show student-initiated tasks increasing from about 20% to 60% and peer group discussion of tasks moving from approximately 3% in traditional systems to 23% for open classrooms for intermediate students.

Among the advantages of open classrooms are: increased student interactions, attention to the individual student differences, flexibility in learning materials and learning rates, and increased student motivation. Undoubtedly this approach will lead to creative designs and further application of the open classroom concept in schools and classes for deaf young people. Criticisms of this instructional approach generally are identified as an increased work load for the teachers, uncertainty that all the content areas have been covered, lack of adaptability in some students, and the need for continuous record keeping. However, this system does encourage the student to constructive, independent action in an area where many deaf children have been thought to be reluctant students. The open classroom is a stimulating environment that, while allowing the student decision-making opportunities, encourages the teacher to motivate students individually. Carefully considered and implemented, open classrooms for deaf students can provide a unique instructional alternative.

Mainstreaming and Partial Integration

Superficially, the concept of mainstreaming and partial integration would suggest that specialists in the education of deaf children would relinquish control of these students to the regular school. Curriculum, therefore, would be solely the responsibility of the regular, public educational system.

Realistically, however, deaf young people still have the same learning difficulties with language, speech, and other areas regardless of the place in which they are instructed. As in the case of open classroom instruction, mainstreaming takes many directions that vary in terms of the length of time, the special supportive services available, and the amount and consistency of instructional management as it relates to deafness. The on-rush of professional articles and the production of how-to-do-it materials strongly indicate that the special educators fully intend to influence the process and content of educational experiences for deaf young people in the mainstream effort (4).

Although there will continue to be those students who adjust with minimum support to the regular school program, two additional thrusts should become more prominent as increasing numbers of deaf children are encouraged to try mainstreaming. The first of these involves a growing use of tutors, interpreters, and other techniques to reduce the usual communication arrangements in the classroom. To this extent, the regular teacher will see the nature of the classroom program altered—an example would be the addition of a teacher of deaf children to an open-classroom setting in the public school. The second thrust should be expected in the parallel instruction for deaf students outside of the regular classroom in order to assure reasonable progress in the integrated setting. An example in this case would involve the partial integration of residential students from a school for the deaf into regular classrooms for hearing students. In this case, the modification to the regular classroom program would be minimal.

The critical observation here is that an increase in the use of mainstreaming by deaf students with quite diverse backgrounds, capabilities, and interests generates a corresponding development, by teachers of deaf children, of techniques for minimizing the effects of conventional mainstreaming procedures for those who need greater instructional assistance. Curriculum changes must either attend to the adaptation problem in the first example or to the efficiency of instruction problem in the second. Partial integration or integration with carefully considered supportive services might seem the direction, therefore, of future innovation.

Educational Technology

The promise of advances in educational levels for deaf students through technology has been illusive. Specific research activities have looked at programmed instruction, media, computer assisted instruction, teaching machines, and many other possibilities. Stepp, a specialist in this area, wrote "I do foresee the day when the master set of instructional materials in the computer will be matched with a major curriculum. At this point in time, we do not have this information" (13).

If the jointure of technology and curriculum is not as yet a fully operating or widespread concept, it is possible to get some idea of the direction and nature of possible interactions. The Callier Center for Communication Disorders (8), for example, has devised a systematic approach to individualizing instruction for deaf children. The resulting profile accounts for "all the variables that are known to affect the learner" and is used to provide both assessment data and base-line data. Curricular activities follow from a prescription developed from this data. Understanding failures, measuring progress, and furthering individualized instruction becomes a part of this program. In terms of curriculum, this model focuses on the learner and the information needed about him but leaves the content free of restrictions. A catalog of materials such as *Materials Useful for Deaf/Hearing Impaired* (10), though not mentioned as part of this data system, might be useful in conjunction with this kind of approach.

Project LIFE (11) materials have gained wide acceptance in schools and classes for deaf students. The Programmed Assistance to Learning (PAL) system enables the students to interact with a filmstrip by using a visually oriented response console. A criterion of 80% correct responses on a filmstrip entitles the learner to move to the next one. A fairly complete instructions manual is included. Although the selection of filmstrips provides an opportunity to meet the child's specific interest, there are limitations imposed by the very nature of the materials and equipment. For example, the content is limited by the availability of filmstrips, and the response is limited to visual recognition.

Other projects involving computer assisted instruction, programmed materials, and similar approaches have also been incorporated into selected parts of the school program. Possibly due to the personal relationships developed between the student and the teacher, and certainly due to the optimum use of teacher aides in many locations, the effect of formally produced educational technology has not always had as profound an effect on classroom activities as might have been predicted earlier. Nevertheless, when the intent of the technology has focused both on the mechanics of instruction and on a consistent learning model, it has produced a more stimulating classroom environment.

In reviewing these projects rapidly, no intent to diminish their considerable significance is inferred. In fact, the current projects are carefully conceived and should lead to even further improvements. Further acceptance of technology in the education of deaf children may have to await a more complete instructional design within schools and classes to fully utilize this potential.

Special Purpose Projects

An alternative approach to curriculum is to set aside the larger objectives of the school and to concentrate on very specific groups of students or on selected subject matter. Instruction of deaf students with additional handicapping conditions (12) has been a productive area. Adaptations of Piaget's developmental theories of intellectual growth have found their way into games and activities which may be used both with and without words to promote thinking skills and social interactions. Interest has also been generated in aesthetic awareness through the arts. Some of these areas are more highly articulated than others, and all of them have been encouraged beyond mere advocacy and have moved forward sufficiently to be included in this discussion of curriculum.

Although programs for deaf students with additional handicapping conditions have existed for many years, the past decade has seen greater efforts in identification of these students, individualized instruction based on better defined instructional objectives, and the application of operant conditioning and experience-based activities. The *Annual Survey of Hearing Impaired Children and Youth* (14) has published data on these young people since 1968 and the *Directory of Programs and Services* (1) of the *American Annals of the Deaf* has relevant summarized data in the 1974 and 1975 editions. Projections through 1980 estimate that as many as 2,000 multiply handicapped deaf persons will reach 19 years of age each year. The program at the California School for the Deaf, Riverside (9), has received particular attention and has served as a model for developments in other parts of the country. The development of communications skills and mathematics and uses of teacher-made materials, team teaching with individual and small groups, and "behavioral engineering" to effect the instructional program are key aspects of instruction for these students. A token-economy and consistent reinforcement of appropriate behavior, both in the classroom and the dormitory, are all integral parts of this instruction. In this illustration, the approach to curriculum has been designed and described as being uniquely appropriate for multiply handicapped deaf students rather than an adaptation of the existing school program; this trend is likely to continue.

Daily living skills ranging from self-confidence to interpersonal relations, from consumer education to health and grooming, have found their way into the curriculum (5, 7). Preparation as a consumer, an employee (other than vocational education), marriage, family, and other life expectancies have developed from informal discussion to some forms of systematic presentation. Within this context, an effort is being made to prepare the deaf citizen for a positive role in community living. This instruction tends to be by practice, example, and direct student involvement.

Another indication of diversity can be found in games and activities that follow a developmental sequence. In the book *Games Without Words* (16) thinking skills are encouraged by activities, including sorting, ordering, classifying, and other attack skills that lead to what might be termed "creative thinking."

The arts have also become a focus of attention for classes of deaf students (15). In a sense, this extension of communication may have special significance for deaf students whose more formal language skills may be less than sufficient, as well as for students who seek to gain a more complete sense of the world around them. These experiences with art form can enhance both the school and out-of-school environment.

Summary

Curriculum development for deaf children has been generated most frequently where simple adaptations from the broader field of education were not sufficient to meet the unique needs of deaf students. Not surprisingly, these efforts are developed most completely in the early school years where speech, listening, language, and cognitive skills need to be encouraged. From this perspective, it would seem likely that early education programs will show a consistent approach based on stated objectives evolving from a central instructional concept. They will not have separate and discrete plans for teaching speech, listening skills, related language skills, cognitive development, and school activities. Instead, the programs will be proposed as integrated units permitting considerable flexibility in the language and subject matter used, but also requiring faithful application of the instructional system.

Open classroom approaches to instructing deaf children have survived the initial adjustments necessary to be effective with them, and this development should show greater variations and increased use in schools and classes for deaf children. In addition to the flexibility provided in the selection of subject matter, the organization of this material can be tailored to provide an individualized approach to learning. Both the content and the process of education can be readily adapted for individual students. Perhaps one of the major benefits, however, results from the independence the deaf child can demonstrate in the open classroom setting. If one of the educational goals for deaf children is to reduce dependence and encourage self-sufficiency, this approach to learning should have significant benefits.

In a similar sense, partial integration of deaf with hearing students and more complete mainstreaming may also encourage responsible and mature approaches to instruction on the part of the deaf student. Though not necessarily desirable for all students, some, perhaps limited, integrative experiences should be beneficial for most. Since partial integration provides greater opportunities for selecting instructional alternatives, it might be reasonable to expect greater expansion in this area than in more extensive mainstreaming. At issue, of course, is the degree to which the expert in deafness is essential to minimize, for the student, the communication problems imposed by deafness and to assist him in accomplishing a reasonable level of academic success. Since the special educator is the prime mover in developing the deaf child's communication skills, it is quite possible that the future will see the development of selective integrative experiences for larger numbers of deaf students while, at the same time, evidencing some retreat from the earlier impetus toward mainstreaming. Mainstreaming will continue, but partial integration should affect a greater number and diversity of deaf young people.

The effect of educational technology on instructional programs for deaf students should continue to develop, although the nature of this change is uncertain. The number of possibilities for using these materials, systems, and devices will grow and the variety of applications should show some creative development.

Finally, the special purpose projects that have been implemented certainly meet their stated objectives. The interest in the arts, in the students with additional handicapping conditions, in skills necessary for living in the community, and in developing thinking skills have resulted in creative, though limited, expansion in schools and classes for deaf students. These projects have yet to be incorporated in broader curriculum planning, but they have presented new approaches and new ideas that should expand to the educational goals for deaf learners. Since these projects do have specific, discrete objectives, they can be carefully organized, implemented, and evaluated. Further development in this area seems highly likely.

This review of curriculum has selected activities currently in progress which appear to be representative of continuing development by educators of deaf children. These benchmarks have been used to project significant instructional efforts for the next few years. Although a reasonable attempt has been made to highlight the direction of discussion and development in curriculum for deaf children, many potentially important programs could not be discussed for lack of space. Many of these programs, because they have definite value in curriculum planning, have been listed and referenced on page 140. The increasing number and variety of these adaptations, in conjunction with the trends discussed above, forecast both systematic and creative progress in curriculum planning and implementation with deaf students.

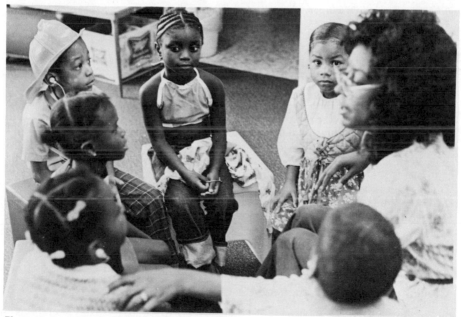

Photo courtesy of Pre-College Programs, Gallaudet College.

9   Richard R. Kretschmer, Jr., Ed.D.

Language Acquisition

Dr. Kretschmer is associate professor of the Department of Special Education and the School of Psychology, University of Cincinnati, Cincinnati, Ohio.

The past two decades have seen an information explosion with regard to the interest in and understanding of the normal language development process, as well as the strategies employed by children in that process. The impetus for this dramatic increase in knowledge has been the interface between the study of child language and the formulation and reformulations that have occurred in linguistics and/or psycholinguistics. As new models evolve in linguistics and/or psycholinguistics, there have been concomitant effects in the examination of child language. This activity in language acquisition has served as a stimulus to reexamination of the language acquisition abilities and/or strategies of hearing impaired children. These most recent research efforts in the area of deafness differ significantly in approach and theoretical orientation from previous study in the field (22). The net effect of this different orientation has been the specification in increasing detail of the language performance of deaf children, detail which suggests to some researchers different acquisition mechanisms for deaf children than had previously been supposed.

Contemporary Child Language Research

The shifting perspective in child language research has reflected alterations in theoretical orientations in general linguistics and/or psycholinguistics. Recently, linguistics has shifted from primary attention to purely syntactic matters to an examination of semantic processing (16, 17, 1, 14, 30, 18, 38, 39), whereas psycholinguistics has shifted its attention from a primary emphasis on surface structure (syntactic) processing to concern with the cognitive bases of language, or more specifically the interface between semantics and syntax (11, 5, 7, 54, 53, 58).

These shifts in linguistics and psycholinguistics have produced at least two types of strategies in child language research: a) descriptive studies, which examined general language performance among or within children, and b) studies in which

60

specific language principles and/or learning strategies were examined in an attempt to specify the process by which children learn language.

Descriptive Studies

The child language research of the mid-1960's produced the "pivot-open class" model for interpreting the linguistic productions of children (11, 13, 46). This approach attempted to explain the language output of children in the two-word stage by postulating a two-category system, namely X words, which had the privilege of occurring in either position in a two-word combination, and pivot words, which were permissible in only one position of any two-word combination and tended not to appear as single-word utterances. The consequence of the pivot open-class model was supposed to be that future language growth was dependent upon a consistent, but predictable, division of these two linguistic categories until "adult" equivalents (grammatical categories) were achieved (44).

In the early 1970's a reexamination of the pivot-grammar position was suggested, based on arguments that such an approach dealt only with surface structure and ignored the linguistic context of the child's utterances (7, 10, 12). It could be demonstrated that children possessed more knowledge of language than merely distributional occurrence of words; that is, the same surface structure, *mommy shoe*, could be shown to represent a variety of deep structures such as actor-action, vocative-command, and possessor-possessed. As a result of this criticism, rich interpretation was suggested as an alternative to the pivot-open approach. Consequently, attention was shifted from concern with surface structures to a focus on deep structure understanding (6, 10, 12).

Child language research presently utilizes linguistic models ranging from the generative-transformational approach (17, 18) to the more radical formulations of case grammarians (14) who are committed to the idea that syntax and semantics are inseparable and that a complete description of any utterance is initially dependent on an examination of its underlying meaning.

Using these various models, several long-term language samples from a small number of children have been subjected to analysis so as to derive statements about normal language growth (6, 8, 10, 12). These studies have tended to utilize a rich interpretation technique; that is, using the immediate environment as a support for determining the intent of the utterances produced so that meaningful emerging grammars can be constructed for the children. Discussions about consistencies that seem to govern semantic and syntactic development as well as presumptions concerning the ties between language and cognitive growth in normal children have resulted.

In general, such studies have been supportive of the notions that: a) children's language growth is highly interwoven with cognitive growth; b) early mastery of language is dependent on the child's successful meshing of nonlinguistic and linguistic experiences; c) the focal point of language growth is the development of semantic categories that are useful in the formulation of connected language; d) early utterances of children represent the merger of key concepts that transcend the specific meanings of particular words used, i.e., actor, action, and object (patient); e) early language combinations seem to be prescribed in number and are common to children learning different languages; and f) acquisition of more complex forms, i.e., negation, seems dependent upon the semantic complexity of the form itself.

Earlier descriptive studies focused on production data. Some investigators have challenged the use of such data to posit statements concerning comprehension, since the processes involved in comprehension may significantly differ from those of production (37, 33). An example of this approach was a recent study which investigated comprehension in four children as a developmental phenomenon, by systematically describing comprehension through well defined testing procedures (33). The findings of this study suggested that: a) these children did not understand as much as was attributed to them by their parents; b) that early comprehension was highly dependent on nonlinguistic events; and c) that although language comprehension differed significantly in many respects from production, there were parallels. Although currently limited in number, such studies contribute insight about cognition's role in language learning and about differences and/or similarities between the development of comprehension and production.

Complementary to the aforementioned investigations, which have centered on the linguistic abilities of young children, there have been descriptive studies of the linguistic usage of children beyond the elementary stage of language development (45, 12, 43). The generative-transformational model has been applied to the description of more complex language with the notion of "restricted form" or systematic deviation from normal adult usage emerging (45). That is, in the evolvement toward complex sentence patterns or adult forms, children produce systematic alterations or restricted form-patterns. Most recently, investigators have concerned themselves with the acquisition of either a circumscribed set of morphophonemic realizations, or the strategies employed in the acquisition of complex sentence-forms such as coordination and embedding (12, 43). In total, these studies seem to suggest that: a) predictable patterns of development can be observed in most children with reference to complex grammatical constructions in language; b) although many language forms are established early, refinement of the system continues; c) establishment of grammatical positions within sentences seems to precede the need to refine the exact details of the linguistic principle involved; and d) the rate and direction of language growth of complex patterns seems to be a function of an interface between the linguistic (grammatical) demands of the principle being mastered, and the cognitive (semantic) understandings required to realize the linguistic principle in meaningful communication.

Experimental Studies

In addition to descriptive studies, researchers have examined dimensions of language learning by use of experimental designs in which variables are externally manipulated (4, 24, 35, 15, 5, 25, 28, 23, 19, 20, 56, 9). Such studies have focused on the development of comprehension strategies, or the specific stages that occur in a limited set of production-data such as question forms or pronouns.

At present, these experiments suggest: a) language development is a complex process involving many different strategies depending on the age of the child, or even the linguistic principle to be learned; b) many language forms and functions are not mastered until the late elementary years or beyond; and c) perceptual/cognitive strategies are often employed to master the grammatical/semantic aspects of more complex forms such as before and after.

Although much has been learned in 10 years about child language, each new discovery leads to new questions and/or the need to reformulate old ideas. In addition to what has been referenced in the preceding discussions, current efforts in child language study are also focusing on the following areas:

• earliest stages of language perception and production, especially neonatal and infant performance (48, 26, 27);

• role of cognition in the acquisition of language, particularly from a Piagetian frame of reference (47);

• variations in rate and style of language acquisition that occur among and within children, as well as factors that can influence such variations (49);

• role of sociologic restraints in the production, employment, and comprehension of specific linguistic rules, and/or categories, by children and adults as they learn from, and interact with, their cultures (36, 31, 29).

Current Language Research with the Hearing Impaired

The study of normal language acquisition has yielded new psycholinguistic information and new research strategies. These have generated interest among professionals within the special field who wish to reexamine the question of language development in the hearing impaired, and by researchers outside the field who wish to verify the notion of linguistic universals, by using a sample of individuals who are as dependent upon visual as on auditory input to achieve language mastery (57).

Research Associated with Education of the Deaf

In the past 10 years, work within the field has focused either on: a) descriptive studies of systematic alterations that may exist in the general linguistic abilities of hearing impaired persons or b) on investigations of the comprehension and/or production of specific linguistic principles by samples of hearing impaired children. Comparison with hearing subjects has also been reported, which gives rise to the question of how the data generated by deaf children should be interpreted. Both written production and reading comprehension have received the most attention in recent research because of the difficulties of understanding and eliciting speech from some deaf persons and because manual means of communication, even within this country, differ radically in content and organization across deaf people.

Cooper (21) used a paper and pencil test modelled after the Berko-Gleason morphological study to investigate the understanding and production capabilities of hearing impaired children ages 7 through 19 years (N=140) and hearing children ages 7 through 18 years (N=176). Although the hearing subjects' performance was superior to the hearing impaired subjects throughout the entire age range, patterns of item difficulty proved to be similar for both groups of youngsters; that is, hearing impaired youngsters found the same rules as difficult to perform as did hearing youngsters. Thus, Cooper interpreted his results as suggestive of delayed language development in deaf children.

Schmitt (55) investigated hearing impaired children's comprehension and production of passive sentences by presenting tasks that required matching reversible passive sentences to pictures, and then by providing opportunities for the subjects to generate passive sentences. His results indicated that deaf children up to 14 years of age were generally unable to comprehend or produce sentences in the passive voice, but by 17 years of age about 60% could comprehend passive sentences, whereas only about 30% could produce such sentences.

Hess (32), in a longitudinal study of the oral productions of a hearing impaired boy and a hearing boy who were equated on the basis of MLU, composed grammars for each child in order to study linguistic growth. She observed no essential difference between the two subjects in the development of underlying syntactic structures, as determined by their ability to perform linguistic operations over the five months of the investigation. When the time-delay factor in the deaf subject's language was controlled, he or she evidenced a sequence of acquisition comparable to the hearing child with two exceptions: a) less differentiation of the subject form-class and b) the more rapid acquisition of a completed negative transformation. At the completion of the study, both children had expanded the noun phrase node to include determiner + noun and modifier + noun, the verb phrase node to include verb + noun phrase, and the notion of sentence to include embedding, the essential operations for generating unique, infinitely long utterances.

Kretschmer (41) examined the written productions of 120 hearing impaired and 120 normally hearing youngsters, 12 through 18 years of age. Data analysis employed the early generative-transformational notions of kernel sentence patterns (60) and transformations upon these kernel sentences, as well as restricted form classification (45). The hearing impaired youngsters tended to produce sentence strings that were less complex than those of hearing subjects and which contained many more restricted forms although no unusual "error" patterns unique to the hearing impaired were observed. For every restricted pattern identified in the writings of the hearing impaired group, there were hearing writers that produced the same types of syntactic restricted forms. Although not a specific topic of the study, there were indications of semantic differences that could argue for differences in language usage between the two groups of children.

Power and Quigley (50), in an extension of Schmitt's study, tested for the comprehension and production of passive voice in 50 hearing impaired youngsters, 9 through 18 years of age. The comprehension tasks consisted of moving toys to demonstrate the action of the sentence, or selecting a picture showing the action of the sentence. The performance task required subjects to fill in sentence blanks with the correct set of passive markers. Significant improvement with age took place on all tasks, but even at 17 to 18 years, only slightly more than one-half of the deaf subjects correctly understood passive sentences and less than one-half correctly produced such sentences. Deaf subjects, even at older ages, interpreted passive sentences in terms of the surface subject-verb-object order of the constituents. Power's subjects scored lowest on a test of agent-deleted passive sentences, somewhat higher on reversible passives, and highest on nonreversible passives. *By* was the only passive marker used by most deaf children. A comparison with data generated from studies on hearing children argued again for the delayed language notion.

Quigley, Smith, and Wilbur (52) administered tests to measure relativization, i.e., the ability to process relative sentences, to embed relative clauses into sentences, and to identify and correct instances of copying in relative sentences such as *The boy who the boy is nice.* This latter phenomenon has been found to be a common occurrence in hearing impaired writings. Four hundred-and-fifty deaf subjects (10 to 18 years) and 60 normally hearing subjects (8 to 10 years) were utilized. The subjects were required to make a judgment of correctness when presented with stimulus sentences, and to generate the correct form when an incorrect sentence was noted. Results from all three tests indicated improvement with age for the hearing impaired subjects. The hearing subjects, although much younger, obtained higher scores on all three tests. For both groups, the position and function of the relative clause determined its difficulty. With medially embedded relative clauses, subjects tended to join the noun phrase of the relative clause with the noun phrase of the main sentence, showing a misunderstanding of the sentence. When conjoining sentences, they omitted co-referential subjects and objects. The possessive-form noun phrases were accepted by deaf children when the possessive form *whose* was the correct form.

Quigley, Wilbur, and Montanelli (52), with essentially the same subjects, investigated grammaticality judgments and production of yes/no, wh, and tag questions. As previously, grammatical sense improved with age for the deaf students, but also as previously, the youngest hearing subjects consistently obtained higher scores than most of the deaf subjects. For both deaf and hearing subjects, yes/no questions were easier to comprehend and to judge the grammaticality of than were wh questions, which in turn were easier than tag questions. The phenomenon of copying was more prevalent among deaf children than hearing youngsters, which caused the authors to argue for the coexistence of normal and deviant rules in the hearing impaired subjects.

In a third study with essentially the same sample, Wilbur, Quigley, and Montanelli (61) examined both grammaticality judgments of unreduced and reduced conjoined structures formed by using and, and the ability to produce conjoined structures by combining sentences that permit the application of conjunction-reduction as well as sentence conjoining. Again, grammaticality judgments of deaf subjects increased with age with almost equal correct choices for both reduced and unreduced conjoined structures. Production of conjoined structures was found to be more difficult than judgments of grammaticality for deaf students. While there was a pattern of general retardation with regard to linguistic judgments or productions for the deaf students, several specific syntactic deviations were found to be peculiar to deaf subjects, and resistent to improvement with age, specifically, object-object and object-subject deletions. Such deviations lead to ambiguous sentence productions such as *The boy hit the cat and ran away*. Divergence in performance between the two groups suggested to Wilbur et. al., as previously, the coexistence of deviant and normal rule systems in their hearing impaired subjects.

Kretschmer (42) in a continuing study of written language, collected compositions from approximately 1200 normal hearing and 1200 hearing impaired school-age subjects. Preliminary findings suggest that, as with Kretschmer's first study (41), the language complexity of the hearing impaired group is significantly lower than that of the hearing group. Analysis of the lexical roles in the base structures of most sentences shows that hearing impaired youngsters even up to 20 years of age tend to focus on the actor/action/patient/location format, with reduced use of process, stative or process/stative verbs. Consistent failure of hearing impaired writers to observe the semantic features which govern grammatical use within sentences has also been noted. For example, some process verbs are infinitive taking, some are participle taking, and some are both. Hearing impaired subjects tend to formulate a two-category system: infinitive taking or both. Verbs that normally take participles only, are usually cast into the infinitive-taking-only category. The preliminary results of this study suggest to the author that there are differences between hearing and hearing impaired writers, but these differences tend to be semantically/grammatically based rather than merely syntactic. In addition, the simultaneous presence of rules that are comparable to hearing children and rules that are not, have also been observed as found by Quigley et al.

Psycholinguistic Research with Deaf Subjects

Recently, researchers from outside of the field of education of the deaf have become interested in the acquisition of "sign language" in deaf children. Impetus for such investigations has come from comprehensive description of sign language (58), as well as the search for so-called linguistic universals that have been postulated from studies of children acquiring a variety of natural (auditory based) languages (57).

Sign language has an internal structure that can be described as using features analogous to syntactic, semantic, and phonological features of spoken language (2, 3). The phonological aspects of language were particularly salient in a series of memory studies in which it was demonstrated that hearing subjects' recall of manual language was dependent on phonological similarity, while deaf subjects' recall was dependent on formational characteristics of the signs themselves, i.e., hand configuration, placement of the hand, and movement from and toward the body (3).

Huttenlocher (34) suggests that because of the unique structure of sign language, certain concepts and/or linguistic units within spoken language systems are neither needed nor necessary in sign language. For instance, because of the spatial nature of sign language, certain spatial notions may be difficult or even irrelevant to encode in American Sign Language, i.e., *above, below* or *beside*. Such a speculation seems to suggest that the semantic bases of sign language could be quite different from that of spoken languages.

Summary

Contemporary research on deaf subjects suggests a few areas of consensus, namely: a) that there is a delay in most deaf children's language performance; b) that reports by several authors have confirmed the pervasiveness of deviant rule-usage in a number of hearing impaired subjects, particularly in the semantic area or with complex sentence patterns; and c) that many convergent language behaviors that improve with age have been also observed. Such conclusions support the notions that the language of hearing impaired persons might best be described as a dialect of English, analogous to any dialect of sociologically or linguistically isolated groups. A dialect by definition is a systematic variant of any natural language that is still mutually intelligible to users of the dominant language, as in this case normally hearing speakers. The exact extent of this dialect, its growth and transmission, must still be ascertained. In understanding the dialectical development of deaf children, particular attention could be paid to factors such as: a) the influence of instructional systems and educational programs that are designed to emphasize the divergence of language learning in hearing impaired children; b) the isolating effects of *congenital* hearing impairment particularly in light of recent reports that discuss the astonishing auditory perceptual capabilities of neonates and infants (26, 48, 27); c) the influence of various communication systems upon each other, i.e., sign language, reading, writing, speechreading, auditory input, or any combination thereof; and d) the possible alterations that occur in the child-parent relationship with the introduction of hearing impairment, alterations that could produce a more devastating effect on the acquisition of any language system by a hearing impaired child than now supposed.

Future Directions for Research

The author sees at least four directions for future research into language acquisition in hearing impaired children:

● First, there is continued need to apply newly developed strategies for studying normal language acquisition to the investigation of language performance of hearing impaired children. Clarification of the precise nature and general problems of language development in this population is imperative, for, if it is found that there are systematic or dialectic variations in deaf children over many investigations, there will be need to reformulate many of the premises upon which most current language curricula are based.

• As the cognitive bases of normal language development are clarified, application of such knowledge to the study of hearing impaired children will become mandatory, first to validate such cognitive organization notions, and second, to assist educators of the hearing impaired in constructing meaningful educational programs that capitalize on the cognitive potentials of any child.

• Application of current research strategies to study the language learning styles of children should also be used with hearing impaired children for both comprehension and production aspects. The questions one might posit at the current stage of knowledge include: "Do hearing impaired children use similar or different language learning strategies when compared to normally hearing children from similar environments?" "Are there differences among hearing impaired children with respect to learning strategies?" "Are these strategies affected by degree of hearing impairment, by use of early amplification, or by other factors?" "Do multihandicapped hearing impaired children employ language learning strategies that differ so significantly from "normal" deaf children as to warrant differential educational treatment?"

• Study of the sociolinguistic aspects of language acquisition has led contemporary researchers to reconsider the effects of parent-child interaction on the acquisition of language forms (49). The introduction of handicap into this relationship has also been found to be predictable. Consequently, there is need to study the interaction of these two factors to enhance our knowledge of how the caretaker-child relationship can be distorted.

In conclusion, traditional research prior to the advent of the new psycholinguistic explosion, gave indication of some differences between the language abilities of hearing impaired and hearing children. Today and tomorrow, there is opportunity to more precisely delineate the nature of these differences with the expectation of developing teaching strategies and/or curricula that will assist the hearing impaired child in becoming a more proficient user of language.

10   *William C. Healey, Ph.D.*

Integrated Education

Dr. Healey is director of School Services Programs at the American Speech and Hearing Association, Washington, D.C.

The current school scene is replete with new terms, each representing concepts and practices that are intended to effect major changes in educational programming; and each implying a far reaching influence on traditional instruction and services, especially for the handicapped. Examples of such terms are "performance contracting," "open modules," "voucher systems," "computer-assisted instruction," "diagnostic-prescriptive intervention," "accountability," and "mainstreaming." Many additional terms could be listed (i.e., "generic specialist"), some of which represent fad, if not folly. Others simply represent new semantics for venerable educational cliches.

Mainstreaming is neither cliche nor fad. For some special educators, however, it is the recently adopted and popularized catchword for the concept of integrated education. Neither the concept nor the practice of integrating handicapped children into regular education programs is new. Birch and Stevens (5), among others, advocated and practiced the integration of handicapped students into regular classes nearly 20 years before the term "mainstreaming" became a new entry in the educational thesaurus. Many of the observations and recommendations that follow result from the author's 18 years of first-hand experience with the pleasures and frustrations involved in securing integrated educational placements, as well as other valid educational alternatives to self-contained special classes for appropriately selected hearing handicapped pupils and the teachers who serve them. Integration is not a panacea; it is not appropriate for all hearing impaired or otherwise exceptional pupils; nor is it a simple procedure to initiate and maintain, even for those pupils who have the potential to profit from such an educational arrangement. To many special educators and parents, it is the preferred placement. In fact, parents often view the moment of integration as the first or most significant sign of success for their child with a hearing impairment.

Mainstreaming, which exceeds but encompasses integrated educational opportunities for the handicapped, has become a nationalized issue and the new ecumenical movement for education (12). Recent advocates of mainstreaming who consider themselves revolutionaries in education for the handicapped need only be tutored in the not too ancient history of segregated programs for the handicapped. Segregation of the handicapped learner occurred for various reasons, most of which can be summarized by lack of accommodation by the regular school environment. Regular teachers were only too ready to have handicapped children removed from their classrooms. The present cry of some special educators to "get the exceptional child back into regular classes" is the direct antithesis of the equally loud countercry of the regular classroom teacher to "get those kids out of my class." Impasse is the obvious outcome when the convictions of each are expressed simultaneously and each remains equally strong. Without competent planning, management, and evaluation, salted with reasonable logic and common sense, such an impasse can be predicted for many school districts in the not too distant future. Fortunately, however, such hard lines have not been drawn between all educators of handicapped and nonhandicapped pupils. Many practitioners among both groups are working cooperatively to achieve successful integration of handicapped pupils into mainstream educational programs (4, 11). These achievements by special and regular educators are being accomplished in spite of the limited knowledge and dearth of conclusive empirical studies that pertain to the performance of hearing impaired pupils in integrated settings.

The Child

School children seem to succeed best where there is an elegant order in the educational environment and where the attitudes, technologies, and the placements are right.

Some educators fear that returning the exceptional child to the regular classroom somehow will dilute educational programs for nonhandicapped children. It is the experience of this author that the "normal" child will not suffer from learning and working with his handicapped peers. The educational program can become disheveled, impracticable, or even paralyzed only to the degree that regular class personnel fail to: a) adopt procedures that accommodate the learning and social needs of each child; b) develop attitudes of acceptance for the child with special needs; and c) receive and utilize competent support of specialists and aides as required. These conditions are needed in educational programs even in the absence of the handicapped child. Therefore, when these accommodations are made for the exceptional child, the majority of the children in the classroom stand to benefit from them as well. The use of precision teaching techniques, more definition and structure for the curriculum, clear-cut expectations and consequences for appropriate performance of staff (teachers and administrators) all hold promise for producing more appropriate learning for most children enrolled in the regular classroom setting. At present, however, we must remain cognizant of the fact that large numbers of children continue to "fail from" or "fail in" regular classes. Many of these pupils have never been labeled as handicapped and have not spent as much as a day in a special class. As a result of receiving the label "failure" rather than "handicapped," many never qualify for special help. Consequently, advocates of integrated education are really asking regular education to finally recognize and act on its responsibility to design unique programs for the individual child, and especially for the child in trouble. Mainstreaming advocates who are unprepared to cope with the pragmatics involved in successfully integrating hearing impaired children into regular classes will soon discover that they are asking regular educators to overreach themselves. Substituting hope in place of working for success will, in most instances, guarantee failure for the children and the integration process.

Educators, confronted with the placement decision to integrate any handicapped child into mainstream educational programs, must be prepared to make a moral and responsible choice. Advocates for the integration of severely hearing handicapped pupils should not substitute cocksure ignorance for thoughtful uncertainty. Given our present knowledge and methodology, some level of uncertainty will be experienced frequently by the educator responsible for the hearing impaired child when he or she decides that the regular class is the most appropriate placement. In such cases, adherence to and attempts to apply the scientific method are prudent justifiable pursuits. Experienced specialists have known for some time that the single criterion of degree of hearing loss is no predictor of a pupil's success in an integrated educational program, nor can the labels "deaf" or "hard of hearing" be used arbitrarily to decide the educational placement (13, 35). The range of critical predictors involves the pupil's intrinsic motivation, personality, cognitive and communicative skills (including speechreading ability), academic or vocational skills, degree of support from the home, creativity and competence in the teaching effort, and attitude of the school population (peers, teachers, and administrators). Unfortunately, several of these as yet cannot be assessed objectively.

Studies summarizing data needed to help professionals make academic placement decisions are relatively few because research data on learning patterns, effective communication modes, teaching strategies, and auditory, language, and speech performance of hearing impaired pupils in regular education programs are sparse (38, 45, 19, 28, 10, 3, 16). In attempting to identify criteria for proper placement, program staff need to amalgamate the more conclusive results of studies on hearing impaired children and apply the findings to the development of the goals and objectives for the program and the children being integrated. For example, the terminology and classification systems used can be a positive or negative influence on the program (29, 39, 14). In addition, it is recommended that the program supervisor and staff develop a system for reviewing, summarizing, and utilizing research available in such areas as cognition (18, 21, 32), language (28, 9), speech production (25, 43), and hearing aids (30, 17).

Certainly, many other categories could be added to the list. For example, information on formal program management and evaluation is important. Also, the influence of social attitudes on the exceptional child's integration into a regular class has been studied by enough investigators to make it clear that no single criterion for a regular class placement will suffice, that competent diagnostic and placement teams are required, and that the receiving school must be evaluated to determine peer and staff attitudes, curricular alternatives, flexibility of teaching methods, and availability of special support staff, materials, and equipment (2, 8, 41, 7, 27, 36). The principles of adaptation and sequenced programming are critical for both the pupil and receiving instructional staff.

The goals of an integration program should remain child-oriented and should include the development of effective communication, advanced academic and vocational achievement, independence, and social sufficiency.

The System

The enactment of statewide compulsory attendance laws between 1852 and 1918 gave the public school system access to handicapped children and, at the same time, often exempted the mainstream system from any responsibility for their education. For example:

Children whose physical or mental condition prevents or renders un-
advisable school attendance or application to study are exempted from
the compulsory education requirement . . .
(Sec. 12152, California Education Code)

All parents, guardians, or other persons having control of a child between the ages of 7 and 16 are required to send the child to a free public
school all day during the school year. The compulsory attendance requirement does not apply to children whose physical or mental condition, as attested to by a physician's certificate, renders instruction inexpedient or impractical.
(Sec. 2702 and 2705 Delaware Compulsory Attendance Law)

Although service increased appreciably between 1918 and 1970, many public
school districts apparently found it inexpedient or impractical to provide instructional opportunities for large numbers of the handicapped. In most states, by 1970,
fewer than 50% of the children needing special services were receiving them and
these services, frequently, were available only in segregated classes, day schools, or
residential facilities (44).

The 1970's will be remembered as the decade that established for the handicapped the "right to education," "due process," "least restrictive placement" and a
national goal of comprehensive services by 1980. Federal court cases, new mandatory legislation, demands for accountability, and increased funding have had
enormous influence on the continuum of programs and services available. State
laws and regulations are being revised that should enable school districts to implement the most appropriate program and personnel utilization-designs possible to
meet the needs of exceptional pupils (1, 20, 26, 23).

The right to education assures that priority in the use of funds will be given to
children not yet served and those not appropriately served, respectively. It calls for
the establishment of instructional objectives and procedures, the elimination of
racial and cultural discriminatory practices, and the provision of specific due process guarantees in matters involving appropriate identification and placement. In
addition, the eligibility age for service is being lowered or eliminated. In approximately 18 states, the child with hearing impairment becomes eligible for services
through the educational system at birth or as soon as hearing loss is detected. Each
of these actions is historic, positive, and worthy of implementation in each state
and local school district.

The last decade has produced ample evidence demonstrating the efficacy of early
services to hearing impaired children and their parents (35). Provision of early
quality services, no doubt, would allow more children to enter and continue in
mainstream educational programs.

The rather recent practice of integrating preschool hearing impaired children into
regular nursery schools and prekindergarten programs appears promising and
merits further emulation and study. Such practices offer opportunities for the hearing impaired child to gain comprehension of spontaneous language and to benefit
early from exposure to numbers of hearing peers. However, such practices must be
accompanied by rigid scrutiny, research, the development of written criteria for
integration, and supportive services by highly skilled educators of the hearing
impaired and nursery school staff. The parents also should become a team member
in this type of integrated program (34).

The "least restrictive" educational environment as identified by law in most
states is supposed to be the regular classroom. This determination assumes, legally,

that an integrated educational opportunity will be made available to any hearing impaired child meeting the school district's criteria for integration. The new era of the right to education, however, has also assumed that the regular educator (teacher and administrator) will be competent and cooperative. Regardless of their competence, experience has shown that some educators express fear of some exceptional children while others simply demonstrate stubborn resistance, whatever their reasons. As a result, collective bargaining agreements governing integration practices are being drawn between special and regular education personnel, contract provisions are beginning to exempt the regular teacher from taking exceptional children without consent, and formulae are being established that reduce the class size according to the number of exceptional children placed in the regular class (4, 31). In one way or another, each of these actions symbolizes the genuine concerns and needs that must be addressed as the educational system establishes standards and policies that will govern mainstream education for pupils with handicapping conditions. The rights of teachers, for example, to the availability of relevant, quality preservice and inservice education, effective professional support, a reasonable class size, and appropriate materials and equipment are yet to be mandated. Unless these details are attended to, the current enthusiasm for integrated programs might be short-lived. On the other hand, parent participation in preschool programs for hearing impaired children has become mandatory in many special schools and clinics. As a result, parents have been conditioned to an intimate involvement with the educational program and consider nonparticipation to be a violation of their responsibility. Such intensive involvement of family members has not been, traditionally, the experience of parents and teachers who have nonhandicapped children in the regular classroom. In fact, the involvement of the regular school parents has too often been passive, infrequent, or even subtly discouraged.

Many parents of hearing impaired children will expect to be involved actively in the educational process when their child becomes integrated into a regular program. Teachers of such classes will need to understand the conditioning that has taken place, the parental expectations, and the best methods for reinforcing and capitalizing on such interest, motivation, and experience. A 15-minute conference twice a year probably will not suffice. The time and activities required for effective parental interaction need to be planned carefully and scheduled wisely.

In fact, careful planning and wise scheduling probably represent two of the most important steps to be taken throughout the educational system to cope with changes required by the new movements toward equal educational opportunity and integrated education. Although some of the issues remain philosophical, most are managerial and financial. In those states and local school districts where the schedules of personnel have been arranged to permit comprehensive planning and program development, many of the managerial problems involving adequate teacher preparation and support, curricular modifications, and pupil and parent counseling and instruction have been reduced or resolved (11, 4). The financial crisis, however, is pervasive. It affects the total educational establishment and even threatens many of the gains that have been made. Certainly, some of the research that should accompany the integration movement, the modifications needed in personnel training, and the pupil and parent support systems envisioned will not be possible without major fiscal reforms. Integrated education, in the absence of qualitative criteria, can be designed with the intent to reduce the cost of educating children with hearing impairment and other exceptionalities. In fact, the promise and expectation of reduced cost served as an argument and incentive for some school systems to implement programs of integration. Such generalizations are premature. Costs of the integrated programs obviously are lower when:

- audiological, vocational, and other services are not provided;
- teachers and clinicians are assigned unreasonable caseloads;
- pupils are seen by the specialists a) too infrequently, b) in groups that are too large, or c) for instructional periods that are too short;
- parent counseling and instruction programs are limited or not provided;
- inservice, continuing education, and consultation time are not commensurate with the needs of personnel;
- staff with limited preparation and experience are employed;
- the necessary materials and equipment are not purchased.

Based on programs visited and/or evaluated by the author between 1970-1975, these conditions describe the state of integrated services in some school districts. Until more school systems apply rigid measures of quality to detailed computations of program costs, the actual cost of integrated versus segregated special educational programs cannot be determined.

The Future

The future in regular education for the child with hearing impairment has and will continue to depend, in great measure, on the educational establishment's success in finally addressing the needs of the individual learner. In many school districts the achievement of this goal will require enormous change. Education has its share of guardians of things as they are, and they practice in both regular and special programs. The fences built by these practitioners constitute some of the hurdles that must be traversed by any advocates for change. Optimism and commitment are requirements for the successful integration of hearing handicapped pupils into mainstream education. If these prevail on the part of both special and regular education personnel, fewer failures will result.

The habits and organized environments of some, if not many, people are difficult to change, but the real alternatives exist now. For example, some schools have reported a reversal of the traditional concept of integration and have enrolled hearing students in special classes for the hearing impaired (11).

Whatever the plan, the successes reported to date from all integrated educational programs have resulted primarily from the ability of the personnel involved to deal with each daily challenge in a logical, detailed, and practical manner. Many of the keys to success appear simple but are only learned from experience. School personnel need to document and report the methods and program designs that work well.

For example, nearly all successful programs stress the importance of:

- commitment by the staff to the "right to education for all" concept;
- relevant, sequential inservice training that truly helps teachers understand and resolve problems involving the pupil, parents, and curriculum;
- strong support by principals for the integration program and a process for matching pupils and teachers;
- specialists who have information, skills, and time to share with the regular teachers;
- a responsive referral system;

- integrating pupils with high probability of success and planning a program for each pupil, initially, that fits into what the teacher is already doing;
- completing all diagnostic assessments and interpreting this information in behavioral terms to the receiving teacher prior to integration;
- giving the teacher and pupil time alone to become conditioned to each other's personalities and communication patterns;
- making certain that the teacher knows how to enhance the pupil's opportunity to hear (through noise reduction and control) and lipread in the class (both the teacher and other pupils);
- helping teachers prepare lessons using media presentations and visual materials that will be an asset for all pupils and especially the pupil with hearing loss;
- implementing parent instruction and participation programs;
- helping the teacher to understand the pupil's hearing aid or amplification unit, its importance and capabilities;
- providing teachers with the opportunity, initially, to administer tests to the pupil with consultation from the specialist;
- reducing class size or providing teacher aides as necessary;
- providing interpreters as required; pupil-partner note takers during oral reports and discussions; written assignments; and opportunities for the pupil to select his own seat and to move his seat as needed to be able to see the teacher and other pupils;
- providing the opportunities for meaningful social interaction so that low status pupils participate in activities for extended periods of time with high status pupils;
- selecting career teachers to avoid turnover, where possible.

Integrated education for the hearing handicapped population also is faced with what some investigators would consider higher order issues for the future. To have a national goal of full, quality services by 1980 is admirable and desirable. Some of the objectives that must be met include the need to:

- establish state and local standards and procedures for planning, managing, and evaluating integrated educational programs;
- develop formal systems for evaluating program and pupil management effectiveness;
- identify competencies needed by personnel providing assessment, instructional, and related services for pupils in the integrated setting;
- plan for and provide increased opportunities for pupils to participate in integrated career education, prevocational, vocational, and technical preparation, and placement programs;
- increase basic research on the prevention and amelioration of hearing loss;
- formalize and objectify selection and placement criteria;
- evaluate programs of professional/paraprofessional preparation (preservice, inservice, and continuing education) to identify effective training models for replication;
- develop projections for training and employing qualified personnel based on analyses of personnel utilization in comprehensive, effective integrated service systems; and needs assessments in districts lacking quality service and instruction models;

- establish uniform procedures or guidelines for assessing actual program costs and determining criteria for judging cost effectiveness;
- conduct research on the methodological techniques used with hearing impaired children and personnel in regular and vocational education;
- assess the characteristics of quality program administration and supervision.

The needs cited above provide some direction for the professionals in establishing short term objectives. In fact, projects in pursuit of meeting these needs are already underway and, hopefully, their findings will lead all of us closer to the 1980 goal. Fortunately, we can approach the future and its goals one day at a time.

During the past five years, the increasing normalization of education for hearing handicapped and other exceptional children has begun to remedy some of the ills resulting from labeling and segregation (37). Regular and special education personnel must in concert fix their attention on the central question of human capability. Creating an environment in which all children can learn requires improved technology strengthened by a more scientific understanding of human potential as well as a realization of the environmental potential. We have come to understand that segregated environments, although sometimes necessary and positive, nevertheless ultimately may be limiting. Therefore, to successfully perceive and to change the environment is liberating. Integrated education could help to break education's moratorium on individual learning. &

11

Donald R. Calvert, Ph.D.

Communication Practices: Aural/Oral and Visual/Oral

Dr. Calvert is director of Central Institute for the Deaf, St. Louis, Missouri.

The single most important improvement in educating hearing impaired children in recent years has been development of a primarily-auditory approach. Described sometimes as the auditory/oral, aural/oral, or the auditory approach, it has begun to be called the "Auditory Global" approach or method (4). Its roots extend deep from the seeds of Itard and others to late in the 19th century when the Viennese otologist Urbantschitsch advocated defining and using whatever remnant of hearing each deaf child had. In the 20th century this idea was brought to the United States, refined and put into practice by another otologist, Max Goldstein, who advocated using the "Acoustic Method" (11). The value of amplified sound as a *supplement* to lipreading and as an aid in developing speech was later demonstrated in a study at The Clarke School for the Deaf and at Central Institute for the Deaf (14). In the 1960's some European scholars suggested using acoustic stimulation as the *primary* input for language development, even for severely hearing impaired children (23), and examples of the approach and its advocacy became prominent in the literature of the United States (13, 18).

The decade of 1965-1975 is marked by the refining and defining of this Auditory Global method. Of course, the development of miniaturized electronic hearing aids was the *sine qua non* which made this new approach possible, but a number of other factors, described below, were important in realizing the value of acoustic amplification.

First, is recognition that the population of children called "deaf" is not monolithic. Annual surveys of the Office of Demographic Studies at Gallaudet College continue to show that about one-half of the children enrolled in classes for the hearing impaired have pure-tone threshold audiograms reflecting hearing levels of 84 dB or better. Over one-fifth have hearing levels of 64 dB or better. Recent investigators (2, 9) have supported the importance of differentiating the severely hearing impaired population by relating their speech production and discrimination abilities to threshold levels. Even when threshold audiograms are similar, important differences in auditory abilities may be revealed by auditory discrimination tests (7) and by diagnostic teaching and observation (17). Indiscriminate use of the generic term "the deaf" may result in a limiting, self-fulfilling prophecy for the hearing impaired child (19, 24). The term "hearing impaired" is now frequently used.

A second major factor in developing the Auditory Global approach has been the contribution of acoustic phonetics to our understanding of speech perception. The presence of important speech information in the lower frequencies, where hearing impaired children often respond to sound, means that such information may be made available to the child through appropriate amplification. The importance of the transitional characteristics between speech sounds to the perception of the surrounding sounds helps explain why we may "hear" the adjoining high pitched consonant because of the direction in which the lower pitched vowel formants are bent, even though the consonant may not be audible. The concept of linguistic and phonetic redundancy, which is that the speech signal contains *more* than enough information for its perception, explains how we are able to understand speech when parts of it are missing. The relation between acoustic phonetics, amplification, and speech production is described by Ling (16).

Understanding of the nature of acoustic speech information and of differences in auditory abilities among hearing impaired children, has led to continued progress in selective acoustic amplification. The use of a single classroom amplifier for all the children in a room ignores important differences. Even differences between a child's two ears may be important, so that routine binaural fitting may detract from discrimination. There is a considerable challenge to the field of audiology to develop an "audiology of profound deafness," which investigates auditory capacities beyond the simple threshold audiogram and relates these capacities to acoustic amplification.

Another important factor which has led to improvement in the Auditory Global method is early and comprehensive intervention. The growth of early education is reflected in the annual reports of programs and classes for children under 6 years of age published in the *American Annals of the Deaf*. In the two decades from 1951 to 1971, the number of programs accepting children under 3 years of age rose from 109 to 369, while programs accepting children in the 1st year of life, absent from 1951 reports, numbered 65 by 1971. While there is no absolute physiological evidence for the effects of early sensory deprivation, there is evidence that delaying intervention is associated with additional learning problems (6), as well as frequent school reports that children who are started on amplification and auditory training very early make superior use of their hearing.

Early and comprehensive intervention is likely to be successful only if there is careful monitoring of auditory stimulation. Monitoring implies a system to see that the child wears his carefully selected hearing aids constantly, that they operate as they were meant to operate, that the "down time" of a hearing aid is minimal, and that excess canal wax or middle ear conditions do not impede the transmission of amplified sound to the inner ear. The most sophisticated process of hearing aid selection, or the most clever techniques for training hearing are confounded when a simple mass of wax blocks the ear canal or the hearing aid battery is dead.

With the growth in popularity of a primarily auditory approach, there has been a reduced emphasis on visual means of developing oral communication. Some variations of the Auditory Global method prohibit, or at least discourage, the child from speechreading during training in an attempt to foster reliance on auditory speech information. Yet, considering that the majority of hearing impaired children with substantial losses need considerable visual information to receive and understand language, we know remarkably little about speechreading. For example the influence of classroom lighting is not well understood. A few studies have been done recently (8, 10), but there is still much to learn about maximum lighting angle, brightness, and shadow. There is a special need to know more about visual processing of a signal changing rapidly in time, and for developing convincing tests of speechreading aptitude and ability. There does not ever seem to have been as much concern about vision and the hearing impaired child's eyes as there has been about his defective hearing. This is especially significant when one considers that the prevalence of educationally significant visual impairments is greater among hearing impaired children than in the general school population (22).

Increasing popularity of the term "total communication" to describe how teachers and children communicate in a school setting reflects an increasing use of manual modes of communication. This supports the need for research on communication through the visual channel, especially for the rate of message transmission, message distortion, and information loss. Simultaneous manual and oral communication, as "total communication" implies, suggests we need to know much more about their differential rates of transmission, and what happens, for example, to the typical rhythm of speech when the speaker accommodates to the slower rate of manual production.

Critique and Comments on Developments

Advocacy of something new often denigrates something older, which it may seek to replace. So it has been with the primarily auditory-approach to communication for hearing impaired children. Many of its advocates have severely deemphasized, if not outright rejected, the now less dramatic and perhaps more demanding visual/oral approaches. Multisensory approaches, which utilize visual and tactile, *as well as auditory information,* have a long developmental history based on teacher experience, including an opportunity to look at the long-term results of such training as observed in the post-school life of the student. It is a sobering thought that several generations of severely and profoundly deaf people successfully learned oral communication either without the help of electronic amplication, or at best as a supplement to visual and tactile information.

If all hearing impaired children could learn oral communication through primarily auditory approaches, there would be little loss in reducing the availability of programs offering multisensory approaches to developing speech. But is this the case? Although there are reports of profoundly deaf children who make surprisingly good use of aural language, there has been no demonstration that the primarily auditory approach works well with all or most profoundly deaf children, or even that it works well with many severely hearing impaired children. This is not to say that it can work *only* with moderately impaired children. My personal observations confirm that it *can* succeed for children having surprisingly severe hearing impairment. But my observations also confirm that it is very difficult to maintain an appropriate overall program and environment for aural development as described by Grammatico (12), and that, even if the program is well maintained, some children will not make acceptable progress in language and speech development when the program is limited to an auditory approach.

If the primarily auditory approach is the *only* approach available for learning oral communication, future generations of hearing impaired children will have lost valuable alternatives. A view into what that future may look like is available in the suggested use of a "deafness management quotient" (5), where the choices available for hearing impaired children are only two: total communication programs or auditory-oral programs. The quotient, derived from a number of factors, but based heavily on hearing threshold level, would be used to decide which of these *two* alternatives would be chosen.

If the primarily auditory approach is the only approach available for learning oral communication, its "failures" will be taken as evidence for failure of oral approaches in general. *The single strand of acoustic pulses of compression and rarefaction of air molecules is to thin a thread upon which to hand the future of oral communication for hearing impaired children.*

Enthusiastic advocacy of something "new" often causes expectancies to rise unreasonably. In our recent history the proliferation of media, use of operant conditioning, and treatment with acupuncture needles are painful reminders of this fact. Advocacy of the "auditory approach," especially linked to advocacy for "mainstreaming," is not likely to escape this trend. To be heard above the hue and cry of our mass media, or above the claims of advocates of total communication, it is not likely that appropriate conditional disclaimers will always accompany reports of results, or, if present, will be heard or not noted. People often hear what they wish to hear, and there is no parent that would not like to hear about a new approach that will bring his child to a higher level of learning and communication. The slogans of "mainstreaming," "total communication," and the "auditory approach" may produce a generation of parents who have some very high expectancies, perhaps higher than our present state of popular educational management is likely to produce in numbers. If this be the case, the disappointment that follows will have a profound effect upon confidence in educators.

To be effective, the primarily auditory approach requires a careful and systematic program of *monitoring* to see that the hearing impaired child gets the best possible acoustic amplification all of the time. *This is easier said than done.* Any school system, mainstream or otherwise, that purports to use the auditory approach to communication should be willing to accept responsibility for maintenance of a conscientious monitoring system for auditory stimulation. Requirements for such a system are only now beginning to be apparent. They go well beyond the initial audiological evaluation and selection of a hearing aid. The Joint Committee on Audiology and Education of the Deaf, sponsored by the Conference of Executives of American Schools for the Deaf (CEASD) and the American Speech and Hearing Association, (ASHA) has promulgated "Guidelines for Audiological Programs in Educational Settings for Hearing Impaired Children" (15). To meet the level of the guidelines, many auditory/oral programs would probably require expenditures for audiology staff and equipment well beyond that presently budgeted.

The American Organization for the Education of the Hearing Impaired (AOEHI) has listed characteristics of an adequate auditory/oral program (1). Routine and frequent examination of the acoustic characteristics of hearing aids, worn daily by hearing impaired children, has been recommended to insure that children are always receiving the amplification that is intended. The state of California is now studying the effects of constant usage on changes in frequency response and distortion of hearing aids. The results may suggest that equipment and staff for acoustic analysis of hearing aids be available wherever there are children wearing hearing aids. Further, when a hearing aid is being repaired, a temporary replacement with the same acoustic characteristics should be immediately available. For the child wearing two hearing aids, this means having a third one always ready to go. Common canal wax build-up or changes in middle-ear impedance from colds (20) can confound the transmission of sound from the most carefully maintained hearing aids. Routine and frequent examination of ear canals and middle ear function should, therefore, be made, as well as routine tests for hearing threshold. Daily listening analysis of the aids of all children should be made by classroom teachers, with swift follow-up by supervising teachers, on-the-spot minor repairs by resident hearing aid technicians, and furnishing of appropriate "loaner" aids when needed. This routine surveillance takes time—time that a busy staff may not be willing to give day-after-day.

When school programs consider themselves "auditory" programs, using primarily auditory means to develop oral communication, but are unwilling or unable to: a) provide a budget for the supporting services needed for systematized monitoring of auditory stimulation; b) take the time to see that the monitoring system works; and c) arrange for appropriate training or retraining of teachers the stage is set for failure and disappointment. The auditory approach is worth making these commitments, but it may be several years before the majority of programs realize that such commitments are necessary.

A Look Toward the Future

In 1969 I made some predictions for the deaf child in the 1970's based on the logical extension of trends then apparent (3). Looking into the future now I shall emphasize three directions that I should *like* to see followed, perhaps to stimulate a self-fulfilling prophecy that they will emerge and grow. These are a continued systematization of the Auditory Global method, expansion of study of the auditory capacity of severely hearing impaired children, and development of wearable equipment for auditory-tactile stimulation. Systematization of the Auditory Global method should include incorporating the guidelines and suggestions that I have discussed above. In conscientious and knowedgeable hands, this approach can be a major help for deaf people.

An important step in the study of auditory capacity was the conference at The Johns Hopkins University in which the participants addressed themselves to the sensory capabilities of hearing impaired children (21). I have suggested the need for an "audiology of profound deafness," which would be directed toward exploring the border between auditory and tactile sensations, toward refining and expanding tests for the perception of speech and speech-like sounds with severe impairment, toward differentiating hearing aids and other amplifying systems on the basis of feedback for monitoring of speech production, toward predicting from psychoacoustic measures the probabilities of a child's future progress with different approaches to development of communication, and toward furthering the interaction between audiologists and classroom teachers for the benefit of severely hearing impaired children. The field of audiology as a whole has not directed itself in this way, but here and there audiologists have addressed themselves to some of these problems. A concerted effort is needed to bring together our scattered knowledge and use it as a foundation for future exploration of the auditory capacity of hearing impaired children.

Developing wearable equipment for a combination of auditory and vibro-tactile stimulation is worthy of attention. Visual sensory aids seem to be going down a blind alley, confined by size and fragility so that devices cannot be easily worn, limited by dissimilarity to the child's own auditory-tactile-kinesthetic feedback system for speech production, and restricted by the rate at which the visual system can receive information compared to the rate of reception of the auditory system. The information of a vibro-tactile receiver, whether on the skin or at the ear, is isomorphic with the auditory-tactile feedback from the child's speech production and can, therefore, complement his own feedback perception. Further, its response capacity can cope with the temporal features of running speech.

What would be useful now is a wearable device that will not restrict ordinary movement of the child, any more than a regular hearing aid, and will not give him unnecessary discomfort. His hands must be free to manage the typical school functions of writing and handling books and papers. He must be free to wear the device in and outside of the classroom, using it most of the day as he might use a wearable hearing aid. Clothing and movement noise must be controlled so that the speech signal can stand out from excess background noise. The device itself must provide useful tactile information without providing so much that it is not discriminable by the child. Then, the system must be tried with a number of children of different ages, with different hearing levels, in and out of classrooms, using connected speech and speech drills, over a long enough period of time so that a sophisticated staff of teachers and researchers can make judgments about its contribution to speech perception and speech production. The interest of speech scientists, psychologists, and engineers in such a device speaks well for the potential of success by this direction of helping develop oral communication for hearing impaired children. ⚖

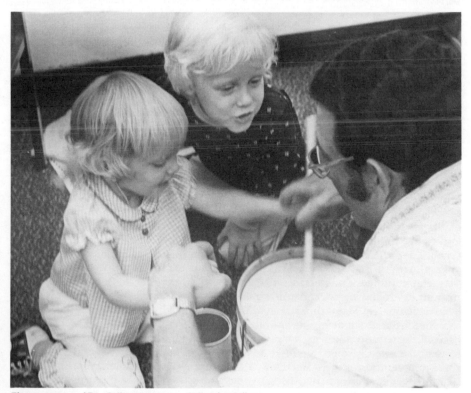

Photo courtesy of Pre-College Programs, Gallaudet College.

12   J. M. Pickett, Ph.D.

Speech-Processing Aids:
Some Research Problems

Dr. Pickett is professor of speech communication research at the Sensory Communication Research Laboratory, Graduate School, Gallaudet College, Washington, D.C.

This paper outlines current developments in speech science as applied to speech communication aids for the deaf and discusses the critical problems for further development of this field.

All of the current aids were designed during the past decade, but their development rests on more than a century of scientific study of speech and hearing, from about 1850 to the present. Alexander Graham Bell was a teacher of the deaf and an applied speech scientist in the first half of this period. Bell's father, Alexander Melville Bell, can also be thought of as an applied speech scientist; he kept abreast of the physics and physiology of both speech and hearing, and he applied this knowledge in his voice training practice. A. G. Bell further exemplified the father's scientific approach; his interest in the telephone originated in his reading of the speech-analysis methods of Helmholtz well before his career in speech for the deaf. The telephone work interacted with his use of a device for speech training of the deaf, in the following way. An instantaneous visual display of speech waves had been developed at Massachusetts Institute of Technology. Bell tried out this display as a speech-feedback device for training deaf speakers. It occurred to Bell that if the "secret" of natural, intelligible speech depended on accurate reproduction of the form of the speech sound waves, then the telephone, to be successful, must preserve and reproduce the speech wave as accurately as possible. From this point, Bell proceeded further by using a physiological model—the ear-drum and ossicles—for designing essential parts of his telephone to change the sound wave into an electrical replica for wire transmission, and then back again into sound waves that had to be as similar as possible to the original wave (36, 4).

Recent research on speech, combined with new electronic techniques, has now

82

produced an advanced technology of speech processing which enables us to analyze and synthesize speech automatically. As these capabilities developed so did the research needed to apply them to alleviation of handicaps of speech communication. Major research questions have been: "Can we develop speech-processing devices that will provide good speech communication for the deaf and hard of hearing?" "Can we build electronic aids to improve the teaching and correcting of speech?" "Can effective artificial speech be provided for persons who cannot speak intelligibly?" and "How can our advanced knowledge about speech be applied to the improvement of hearing aids?"

Certain issues in this field will be discussed in this chapter from a critical point of view. First are characterized the major types of communication problems that need to be alleviated through speech-processing aids; some of the devices currently under development or test are cited. Hearing aids, as such, are not discussed but the reader should especially see references (44, 57). All research activities are not described; these have been covered in recent reviews (29, 47, 27, 41) and in published proceedings of conferences (30, 54, 14, 15, 46). After characterizing the various speech-processing schemes, certain general problems for the field, inherent in the nature of speech and sensory systems, are discussed and speculations are made about the optimal solutions. Finally, research on speech feature discrimination by the hearing impaired is discussed as it relates to perception of speech through hearing aids.

The communication goals to be met by speech-processing aids are: a) speech reception for hearing impaired persons, b) speech feedback for hearing impaired and speech handicapped persons, and c) effective speech synthesis for use by the speech handicapped. These are discussed below.

Speech-Processing Aids to Speech Reception

Visual and tactile transforms of speech have been studied as aids for the deaf since the 1920's, when the advent of electronics made possible the instantaneous frequency analysis of speech sounds. Currently, the prototype aids employ frequency analysis, zero-crossing analysis, and digital processing of speech. The analyzed information is presented to the user by a sensory display. Tactile displays have the advantage of being able to be worn under clothing and they do not require the user's visual attention, an important point if an aid is to be used for deaf infants. The advantage of visual displays is that visual stimulation is better understood than tactile; furthermore, visual speech patterns can easily be portrayed for training purposes by sketches, photos, or overlays. Another kind of presentation is through hearing; however, the sound patterns must be transformed in some manner deemed to improve perception by a hearing impaired person. The advantage of this approach, which we will call auditory recoding, is that speech is normally received by ear, and, with conservative transforms, the method might minimize the problems of learning to perceive speech in terms of totally new sensory patterns.

Current aid designs employ one of four different approaches to the speech-reception problem:

Spectral Method. A set of filters, or other spectrum-analyzing circuitry, continuously derives data about the amplitude-frequency patterns of the sound received. These patterns are presented on an array of visual or tactile stimulators. Examples of systems using the spectral method are the Bell Labs Visible Speech Translator (51, 24) and the Tactile Vocoder (45, 49, 28, 12, 22).

Feature Method. A processed version of the spectral information is presented, attempting to emphasize those sound features that correspond to important articulatory features of speech, such as stop, fricative, nasal/nonnasal, and voiced/unvoiced. These features are very difficult or even impossible to identify by lipreading. Examples of feature-displaying systems are the visual Upton Eyeglass Speechreader (48, 21) and a tactile system tested by Miller et al. (39).

Lip-linked Method (Cued Speech). This method presents code symbols for speech-sound groups that require lipreading for resolution within the group. For example, for one symbol a consonant group is [sh, r, l] and a vowel group is [ee, oh, ah]; this symbol thus defines nine consonant-vowel combinations [shee, shoh, shah, ree, roh, rah, lee, loh, lah], among which the lipreader can distinguish. A group does not represent a sound-pattern code that can function without any other sensory input as can the displayed patterns of the spectral method and feature method. Because each symbol represents a consonant-vowel combination, the rate of symbol presentation is lower, on the average, than for the feature method, but the number of symbols is greater (8 vs 5 or 6). There is one lip-linked system under test—Cornett's Automatic Cuer (6).

Auditory Recoding Method. Automatic frequency division is one method of auditory recoding that tries to take advantage of the ability of the auditory system to normalize the frequency patterns of speech, as is done when perceiving the speech of small children vs women vs men. Roughly speaking, the frequency patterns of women are about 20% lower than those of children, due to the size factor of the vocal passages, and a similar ratio exists approximately between women and men. Hearing impaired persons often have better mid-frequency hearing than high-frequency, and better low-frequency hearing than mid-frequency; they often report that men are easier to understand than women and women than children. A study of hearing aids found male speakers to be much more intelligible than female (38).

Electronic systems that provide adjustable frequency division in real time are now available. The amount of frequency division that should be used may depend greatly on individual hearing characteristics. A recent study of moderate amounts of frequency division showed improved word reception only for a few of the listeners and for only a limited number of experimental conditions (56, 37).

Transposition to the low frequencies of a limited high-frequency region (above 4000 Hz) is a second type of auditory recoding. Tests of this method showed improvements in fricative consonant reception (17, 25).

Radical auditory recoding has not generally proven to be advantageous (50, 35).

Speech Feedback Aids

Feedback of speech is important in the acquisition and maintenance of speech skills. Effective feedback might enable a deaf infant to develop speech, and for persons deafened later in life, it could serve to maintain the quality of speech. The speech reception aids above may also function in monitoring one's own speech, but many of the above systems were conceived especially as wearable speech-reception aids. In addition, special speech-teaching or correcting aids have been developed. The speech analysis principles are the same as for reception aids. Both spectral and feature methods have been used. The displays are visual except for one tactile voice-pitch display (60). Teaching aids can use sensors that are held on the throat to monitor the voice pitch and the glottal action on voiced consonants vs unvoiced consonants (42, 16). Similarly the nasal/nonnasal feature can be sensed by an accelerometer placed on the side of the nose.

Examples of speech feedback aids are the spectrum analyzer LUCIA and a set of pitch, nasality, and S-indicators (1), the voice-pitch trainer FLORIDA (53), and a TV-based system (5). One system under test provides several of the above indications (separately) for computer-controlled training programs (41).

Speech Synthesizers for the Handicapped

Speech synthesis from a phonetic symbol input (synthesis by rule) has been under research and development since the late 1940's, as a means of studying the basic nature of speech communication, and for application to book reading for the blind (43). Speech synthesis may also prove to be an aid for the speech handicapped. Some initial test-uses of a computer-controller synthesizer for neurologically mute persons are under study (13).

Persons with profound deafness of early onset often fail to acquire speech that is intelligible to a normal listener. However, speech training of these persons may develop fairly stable articulatory patterns that are recognizable by a special speech recognition machine (23, 40). This, together with a synthesizer, would provide communication with normally hearing talkers. Much would depend on how many recognizable utterances the deaf user could produce and on the degree to which his correspondents could constrain their own vocabularies to keep within what the recognizer had been taught. Also the number of correspondents would have to be limited and their versions of the vocabulary would have to be known to the recognizer.

The Problem of the Speech Code

Thus far the success of visual and tactile speech aids, and of radical auditory recoding, has been rather limited. Perhaps this is because most of the experiments have not employed efficient training that extended over a period of years (12). On the other hand, one can argue that, to be widely adopted, speech-processing aids should not require such extensive training. Ideally, they should work well without undue learning effort. In order to develop such optimal aids we must take into account certain basic aspects of the problem that are inherent in the nature of speech communication and sensory perception. These problems have to do with the speech code and perceptual organization.

The nature of the speech code is a major difficulty. Consider that the slow progress with speech aids stands in marked contrast to that of the useful Optacon tactile print reader for the blind (55). There has been much more research effort on speech aids than on print-reading aids for the blind. I think this discrepancy in speed of development is due largely to the highly encoded nature of speech. Unlike printed letters, the code of speech is not alphabetic. Each unit of speech is encoded in terms of the identity of adjacent units and in terms of the stress-intonation patterns of the language. Thus the perfect decoding of any stream of speech must be a very complex process. Intensive research is being carried out on this problem and progress is being made (23, 40).

Some Speculations on the Perceptual Problems

Speech behavior probably evolved biologically, together with auditory mechanisms that became specialized for speech perception. Recent findings in anthropological phonetics suggest that socially effective vocal anatomy is responsible for the evolution of human speech (34). In addition, there is evidence that the auditory system possesses innate sound pattern detectors that are specific to human speech features (11). Human hearing may be highly specialized for speech perception (32, 31). Similarly the patterns of speech may have been functionally selected in evolution to match auditory capacities. Hearing and speech together form a highly robust system of coded communication that is capable of almost infinite flexibility of reference and meaning, and this may be due to a highly specialized evolution.

Visual and tactile aids may encounter serious interfacing problems due to biological incompatability with the speech communication system. Indeed vision and manual touch have probably evolved their most salient perceptual features to function optimally for behavioral demands that are not at all related to the spoken language system. This is not to say that visual and tactile speech aids cannot alleviate speech communication problems, but I think we should view the field with a healthy respect for the nature of man and his language mechanisms instead of assuming that man possesses a sensory learning system with unlimited capacities that may be used in any desired way.

Human sensory systems appear to be naturally designed to perceive object constancy in the external world, despite changing stimulus patterns (20, 19, 18). What are the object constancies of speech? I believe they are the articulatory patterns. If this is true, a speech aid should try to present stimulus patterns that are interpretable on a constancy principle. Examples already exist in two useful natural-aid systems—visual lipreading and the tactile Tadoma method—that sense articulatory patterns rather directly.

Visual information about some aspects of speech articulation is available on the face of a speaker. This enables lipreading to contribute to speech reception by hearing impaired persons and by normally hearing persons in noisy situations. However, there are important articulations of the tongue, velum, and glottis that are not visible, and this imposes severe limits on lipreading. On the acoustic side, the patterns of speech have no simple relations to the articulatory patterns. Nevertheless, for truly effective aids we may need to decode from acoustic to articulatory terms (32, 31).

These considerations also apply to tactile aids. Deaf-blind "listeners" are sometimes able to receive speech to a useful degree by feeling the speaker's lips, jaw, and larynx (Tadoma method) (2). Here, as in lipreading, the articulatory information is directly available. Are there other tactile patterns that would have constancy properties corresponding to articulatory constancies?

The salient perceptual characteristics of touch are not very well understood. Active touch on an object normally functions together with movements of the hands (20, 19, 18). Even passively received touch usually involves a movement of the stimulating object across, or taps to and from, the skin. Vibration is passively sensible by touch but rarely used functionally. Human touch probably evolved primarily to function as part of kinesthesis. There are also kinesthetic aspects to speech (3), so it would seem that an optimal tactile speech aid should employ kinesthetic stimuli. The Tadoma method apparently is substantially kinesthetic. The tactile vocoders tested thus far have employed only passive tactile reception.

Auditory speech-processing aids, such as frequency dividers and transposers, should be designed to provide auditory patterns that are articulatorily possible in order to take advantage of the articulatory constancies that we presume to operate in the hearing system for speech.

Speech-Feature Discrimination as a Description of Residual Hearing

Speech science has provided us with detailed acoustic descriptions of the essential sound patterns, or acoustic features, of speech. These features are the vowel formants and their transitions, the noises of fricative and stop consonants, and the temporal pattern of sound. Recently, certain investigators have studied the discrimination of such speech features by hearing impaired listeners (7, 8, 9, 10, 58, 59). This research has employed two new methods: a) the use of synthetic speech stimuli with controlled variation of the acoustic features, and b) analysis of listeners' responses to spoken words to reveal the feature dimensionality of the impaired listener's speech perception and his lipreading.

These studies have provided a deeper knowledge of the auditory nature of the speech discrimination problem of the individual hearing impaired person. In fact, a major finding is that individuals vary a great deal in their auditory capacity to discriminate the acoustic features of speech, and in ways that cannot always be predicted from information on the pure-tone audiogram. In some individuals the low-frequency part of the vowel spectrum (first formant) has been found to interfere with discrimination of an important feature that is higher in frequency; and this interference may be relieved by partial suppression of the low-frequency sound. Findings of this type have a great potential for application to the fitting of hearing aids and the design of auditory training material. The use of synthetic speech stimuli in diagnosis and therapy is now highly feasible, but awaits the necessary test development and clinical-therapeutic demonstrations of effectiveness.

Further Development and Research

The usefulness of speech synthesis to handicapped persons depends on the trade-offs between convenience, cost, and speech-processing technology. These can now be determined through field-testing programs in which prototypes or simulations are used (43).

Research for speech-processing aids to reception and speech production can also benefit from field testing, but, because of the problems inherent in transforms of speech as noted above, results may often be only a little encouraging and progress may be slow.

Basic research on tactile stimulation and perception is needed. Communication by the Tadoma method should be studied. Visual codes should be developed that employ highly salient visual features for the indication of speech features.

Training procedures and situations must be optimized, giving special attention to the feedback conditions for speech training and correction (52).

Clinical adaptations of speech feature discrimination tests need to be developed and tested for use in the fitting of hearing aids and auditory training therapy.

Note: The sections of this paper on speech-processing aids and their problems appeared as a chapter in *The Nervous System*, Vol. 3, *Human Communication and Its Disorders*, D. B. Tower, (Ed.), New York: Raven Press, 1975, commemorating the 25th anniversary of the National Institute of Neurological and Communicative Disorders and Stroke, and the preparation of these sections was partly supported by that Institute.

13

Mervin D. Garretson, LL.D.

Total Communication

Dr. Garretson is assistant to the dean for planning/dissemination, Pre-College Programs, Gallaudet College, Washington, D.C.

In brief historical perspective, the concept of total communication has its antecedents in the early 16th century. The first recorded statement that the deaf could indeed be taught a language was made by a 15th-century humanistic educator, Rudolf Agricola, in *De Inventione Dialectica*, published posthumously in 1521 (4). This observation, revolutionary for its times, received currency from the Italian, Girolamo Cardano, generating a flurry of activity in creating a number of methodological artifacts for the instruction of deaf children and adults. In rapid succession followed the pioneering accomplishments of Ponce de León, Dalgarno, Bonet, de Carrion, and Pereira, each claiming and apparently demonstrating spectacular success from a progression or combination of mimetic gesture, fingerspelling, signs, and speech (4, 13).

These early master-teachers generally operated with selected students in a tutorial rather than classroom setting. It was not until the 18th century, with the advent of schools and regular classes for all deaf children, that a polarization developed between manual and oral techniques. With the increased number of students and consequent growth in class size, the French Abbe de l'Epée felt time limitations precluded a dual method approach—development of language and learning, and, at the same time, speech. His choice was a noncompromising manual method. The German oral teacher, Samuel Heinicke, took a diametrically opposite approach, and the either-or controversy began in earnest.

Over subsequent years the manual-oral pendulum swung back and forth, with an occasional merging of the two methodologies for a combined approach. In 1880 the oral movement gained renewed and long-lasting impetus on the continent with adoption of a series of pro-oral resolutions at the International Conference of Teachers of the Deaf in Milan, Italy (4, 13). Meanwhile, a majority of American state schools committed themselves to oral-only approaches in the primary classroom but continued a permissive communication methodology at the middle- and upper-school levels. However, most private and parochial schools, day classes and programs, and a smattering of residential schools maintained an exclusive oral philosophy.

During the 1950's a segment of the profession began to articulate the need to develop a philosophical framework that would recognize the value of manual modes as useful adjuncts to accepted aural/oral approaches. Emphasizing the need for all avenues of visual reinforcement, concepts like multi-communication and the need for multiple communication skills began to appear in print and as part of discussions with parents and within such allied disciplines as rehabilitation, religion, psychology, and audiology. Although occasional reference had been made to "total communication" in dance and theatrical circles, its coinage with application and widespread usage with the deaf began in the late 1960's when a deaf educator and parent of two deaf children, in a moment of serendipity, came up with the terms "total approach" and "total communication." Roy K. Holcomb, during graduate study at the leadership training program at California State University at Northridge, continued to pursue adoption of these terms as a means of articulating such a flexible approach. In 1968, upon becoming area supervisor of the Santa Ana, California program for the hearing impaired, he was instrumental in achieving formal acceptance of total communication as the philosophy of the school (14).

In recent years, a number of efforts have been made to reach consensus on an acceptable definition of total communication. Regardless of the sometimes hairsplitting semantic and theoretical differences among definers, explicators, and discussants, a pervasive stream of agreement appears in these salient assumptions: a) the concept as a philosophy rather than a method; b) a combining of aural/oral-manual modes according to the communicative needs and the expressive-receptive threshold of the individual, and c) the moral right of the hearing impaired, as with normally hearing bilinguals, to maximal input in order to attain optimal comprehension and total understanding in the communication situation (9, 14, 15, 16, 20).

Communication has been described as linear when a sender attempts to transmit a message over a selected channel to a receiver, as in television commercials, prepared talks, and in other instances when the receiver or audience may be essentially nonparticipatory. However, interpersonal communication is primarily circular rather than linear, a meeting of minds occurring between sender and receiver in encoding and decoding messages. Speaker and listener switch roles in a continuing dialogue, effecting a sharing of ideas and feelings that results in change and interaction for both. It is talking with people, not at them. John Dewey has defined communication simply as participation. Ben M. Schowe, Jr., an English teacher at the Model Secondary School for the Deaf in Washington, D.C., suggested to an in-house school committee on communications improvement that communication is a highly idiosyncratic matter and that choices of modes by senders are influenced by their own skills as well as the skills of the receiver and the nature of the communication situation, be it informal—one to one, or highly formal—one to many. It is inclusive rather than exclusive and avoids value placement on any selected mode and acceptance of whatever the receiver/sender finds adequate for real communication. This kind of circular, nonmanipulative communication tends to be nurtured and enhanced in an atmosphere where communication needs and objectives hold first priority.

Some years back Mary E. Switzer, then administrator of the Social and Rehabilitation Service, observed that educators and others concerned with the growth and development of hearing impaired children have sometimes appeared to be more concerned with methods and theories of communication than with encouraging communication itself. She stated: "Communication is a subtle thing, for it is not words only, not seeing only, not hearing only, not spirit only, not always direct confrontation—but all of these. How do we use what *we* have to bridge the gulfs in our society today?" (27). A basic premise of total communication is that the strengths in one mode are utilized to reduce weaknesses in another mode—that they are mutually reinforcing. At a Center for Applied Linguistics (CAL) conference in 1970, linguists were intrigued by the fact that in using two discrete languages, such as French and English or any other paired dichotomy, it is not possible for a bilingual person to use both languages simultaneously, but with a signer-speaker "it is possible to utilize the unique relation of simultaneous systems for mutual reinforcement" (25).

From the foregoing rationale it may be perceived that total communication is neither a method nor a prescribed system of instruction. It is a philosophical approach that encourages a climate of communication flexibility for the deaf person free of ambiguity, guesswork, and stress. It acknowledges the fact that the hearing impaired require a totality of visual support. Hierarchical distinctions among the various modes are avoided; each modality receives legitimate status as an acceptable instrument for human interchange. In addition to an educational staff with professional preparation in administrative, instructional, auditory, and counseling theory, including up-to-date techniques and strategies in subject matter presentation, I believe that some assumptions and principles requisite to an effective total communication program include:

- Acceptance of the underlying philosophy that all visual, manual, oral,and auditory roles in the communicative process are complementary, including administrative support and commitment to total communication, in theory as well as in application;

- Early identification and full acceptance of the child as a hearing impaired individual by both the parents and the school, since learning occurs best in an atmosphere of ego development and self-concept; this includes recognition of the need to begin when the disability is first diagnosed in order to provide for immediate communication, learning, and language development;

- Belief that increased learning potential is achieved with the added dimensions of a multisensory approach, particularly in group situations; provisions for individualized communication strategy by allowing for the different levels of ability in the various modes of communication; increased likelihood of incidental learning, particularly when teachers and staff members utilize all modes when communicating among themselves in the presence of a deaf child;

- Provision for communication training as an integral part of the staff development program, including skills in amplification, manual, and speech/lipreading approaches, and

- Awareness of the implications for total communication beyond the classroom, which involve social and cultural, as well as instructional, interchange, and which bear relevance to variations among user- and teacher-roles, as in personal counseling, peer interaction, and simple chitchat; recognition of carry-over into after-school life, such as the ability to use both oral and manual interpreters in a variety of settings; and provision of opportunities for a wide choice of social communication with both deaf and hearing persons.

Observing the dictum that a good definition needs to be brief, the most recent Conference of Executives of American Schools for the Deaf committee to define total communication proposed the following dictionary definition at the meeting of the CEASD at Rochester, New York, May 1976, "Total communication is a philosophy incorporating appropriate aural, manual, and oral modes of communication in order to ensure effective communication with and among hearing impaired persons."

Elements in the total communication process fall into two general categories—manual and oral. In other sections of this Bicentennial monograph, detailed material is presented on aural/oral methodology. With mushrooming interest and study in the last 10 years from linguists, sociologists, psychologists, and educators in the characteristics and possibilities of sign, a number of modified or new systems have developed that lead to further sub-grouping within the manual spectrum. Space does not permit a detailed analysis of each system, other than a brief introduction and identification of primary sources. Some total communication programs have opted for a specific manual system, but practically all of these recently developed manual complements have borrowed their basic vocabulary from American Sign Language (ASL).

It is generally recognized today that American Sign Language represents a formal language structure distinct from English, with its own semantic, syntactic, morphological, transformational, and phonologic rules—the latter constituting cheremes rather than phonemes (2, 3, 8, 10, 23, 24). Cheremes are defined as the four parameters of signs—configuration, movement, orientation, and place of contact. When combined simultaneously, they form the sign vocabulary according to formational rules that are specific to each sign language, e.g., ASL, Iranian Sign Language, or Japanese Sign Language. Sign symbols, like word symbols, express the thoughts and ideas of the signer. ASL has as many idioms as spoken language and is no more "concrete" or "conceptual" than spoken language. Minimal fingerspelling may occur within this system.

Sign English (Siglish) is perceived as an ASL-based approach moving along a continuum toward the syntax and word order of English with increased use of fingerspelling rather than invention of new signs for inflection, affixes, and the like. Siglish may be used simultaneously with speech and may be viewed as the manual component of what is also known as simultaneous communication. It continues to be the standard mode utilized by most deaf adults today in this country with a working knowledge of both English and ASL-based signs.

Manual English, while retaining many of the root signs of ASL, has attempted to devise some new signs or to modify existing signs in the various systems, Signed English (5), Seeing Essential English (1), Signing Exact English (12), and Linguistics of Visual English (31). Manual English attempts to reproduce English morphology in a visual mode with varying principles established for syllabic or morphemic distinctions by specific rules for movement, use of compound signs, or other criteria, which distinguishes the different systems. Generally the new sign systems have created signs for affixes, verb endings, plurality, articles, and English words previously having no sign equivalent, including italicization for groups of words with a basic ASL sign, e.g., the words *lane, road, street,* and *path,* which retain the same movement but begin with an 1, r, s, or p handshape to identify the specific word. The objective of these systems is to provide in signs another code for visual representation of English. When used in combination with aural/oral modalities, it is anticipated that multiple reinforcement of the English language is effected.

The gestemic classification may be self-explanatory as referring to communicating without a formal language. "Childrenese" develops out of ad hoc, short-lived signs used by young deaf children, much like baby-talk. Esoteric signs, sometimes used interchangeably with childrenese, signify in-group signs developed within a certain school, program, or geographical locality and understood chiefly by this

---

Elements of Total Communication*

American Sign Language (Ameslan or ASL)
standard signs   unique grammar
non-English language   unique syntax
some fingerspelling
          one sign = one concept

Aural/Oral
amplification   oral gesture (silent mouthing)
lipreading   speech
cued speech (eight hand configurations, four facial positions)
          one lipsign = one or more phonemes

Fingerspelling
finger rather than hand signs
letters run together as in oral or written production
Rochester method (fingerspelling combined with speech)
          one hand configuration = one letter

Gestemic
childrenese   natural gestures
esoteric (localisms)   pantomime
international sign
          one gesture = one concept

Manual English
Seeing Essential English   fingerspelling
Signed English   standard sign often used as root
Signing Exact English   creation of new signs for inflections,
Linguistics of Visual English   endings, tense, affixes, articles
          one sign = one word or affix

*Siglish (Sign English)***
Pidgin Sign English   standard sign modified on con-
fingerspelling   tinuum toward English
syntax heavily English-   gear-shifting between English and
   oriented   ASL idiom
          one sign = one concept

---

*Note: In development of this chart reference was made to the work of Dennis Cokeley of the Kendall Demonstration Elementary School and Roslyn Rosen of the Model Secondary School for the Deaf in precollege programs at Gallaudet College.
**Bernard Bragg of the National Theatre of the Deaf uses the term "Ameslish."

small group of users—a kind of dialect apart from ASL. However, it should be observed that when used in conjunction with speech and lipreading it is possible for most signers to follow fairly well. I have previously discussed international signs as a form of "pure" communication with iconic properties that transcends formal language barriers, and hence, a nongrammatical and nonscientific means of sharing and communicating thoughts (11).

Fingerspelling is simply producing on the fingers of one hand (in the British Empire, on two hands) a letter by letter representation of English or other foreign words. Known as the "Rochester method" when used in combination with speech, fingerspelling utilizes a different hand configuration for each of the 26 letters of the alphabet (22).

In preparation for this paper, an information questionnaire was mailed to the 145 educational programs with a minimum enrollment of 100 each, representing a total of 35,119 students, as listed in the 1975 *Directory of Programs and Services* published by the *American Annals of the Deaf*. In addition to questions about the incidence of total communication, information was requested from each program on definition of the term, date the philosophy was adopted, significant positive or negative changes observed in speech, English, overall communication, self concept, affective growth, and finally, comments and prognosis for the next 10 years. A total of the 122 responses received yields the following breakdown:

Significant positive, negative, or unchanged/uncertain changes noted since adoption of the total communication philosophy (107 programs reporting)

	Positive		Negative		Unchanged/ uncertain	
	Programs	%	Programs	%	Programs	%
Speech	54	51.9%	12	11.2%	41	38.0%
English usage	79	73.8%	2	1.8%	26	24.3%
Overall commu- nication	81	75.7%	4	3.7%	22	20.5%
Self concept	87	81.3%	1	0.9%	19	18.0%
Affective growth	78	72.8%	1	0.9%	28	26.0%

A substantial number of programs reported that although they had used a flexible communication approach for years, total communication has not, as yet, been adopted as a philosophy for the school. Seventy-six programs listed dates of adoption (Figure 1).

A great deal of similarity was reflected by the definitions presently functional in the various day and residential programs. A preponderance of positive and enthusiastic comments were recorded, covering a broad range of individual opinion and prognosis for the next 10 years. However, a number of concerns were consistently expressed. These may be summarized as the need for: a) a single, standardized sign system; b) continued research and study with appropriate measuring instruments for objective and rigorous documentation of results, and c) more effective implementation of the aural/oral component of total communication. An overwhelming percentage of the respondents predicted continued momentum for the total communication philosophy, with only two responders specifically forecasting disenchantment with the approach over the next 10 years.

Figure 1.   Growth of programs officially adopting total communication as an educational philosophy in communication since 1965-1966 (76 programs responding)

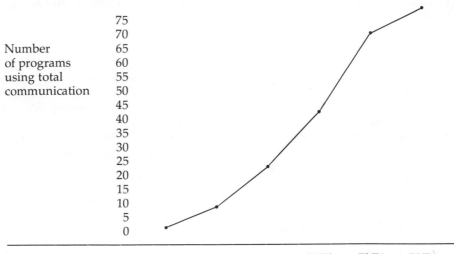

Number
of programs
using total
communication

75
70
65
60
55
50
45
40
35
30
25
20
15
10
5
0

65/66   67/68   69/70   71/72   73/74   75/76
School-year in which philosophy was officially adopted

Number of programs adopting total communication: 107 (87.7%)

Throughout preschool to graduation	76
With options for separate aural/oral or total communication track	18
In upper school only	4
New program, full implementation in 1976	3
Flexible approach but not fully total communication	3
Adopted for multiply handicapped	2
Used on prescriptive basis (oral school)	1

Number of programs that have not adopted total communication: 15 (12.3%)

Strictly aural/oral approach	12
Rochester method	2
Speech clinic (not a school program)	1

It is difficult to identify and assess the significance of developments over the last decade that may have contributed to the widespread acceptance of total communication. In addition to the desire for continued improvement of the status of education of the deaf and the constant search for more effective techniques toward excellence, major influence may have come from these related events:

● The rise of consumerism in the United States with its resultant spillover into the field of deafness, which encouraged parent and adult deaf input; heightened sensitivity to minority groups (30); involvement of the deaf community in policy and decision-making through participation in teacher preparation programs and seminars and workshops sponsored by the Rehabilitation Services Administration under the dynamic leadership of Boyce Williams and Mary E. Switzer, the Bureau for the Education of the Handicapped, including Media Service/Captioned Films, and other branches of the Department of Health, Education and Welfare, and similar activities at the state and local level; the growing number of deaf persons at management levels in education, government, industry, and organizational work, which, with the invention of the teletypewriter terminal unit by Robert Weitbrecht and captioned and interpreted TV programs, have contributed to increased independence and visibility for the deaf person.

● Prolific research and studies into sign phenomena and its application to early language and social development by linguists, sociolinguists, and psycholinguists (28, 29, 17, 3, 18, 23, 24, 21, 8); and parallel research and study by educators of the deaf (7, 6, 26).

● Expanded organizational and institutional activities, including the proliferation of postsecondary junior college and vocational-technical programs, which have all contributed to a sort of information explosion. Included would be all of the national organizations initially involved in the now defunct Council of Organizations of the Deaf.

● Sign language awareness and interest as demonstrated by the National Theatre of the Deaf, the spectacular increase in manual communication publications by the National Association of the Deaf's Communication Skills Program, course offerings in teacher preparation centers and regular school curriculums.

Finally, as a profoundly deaf individual who values both manual and oral communication skills, I share the concerns expressed by many who responded to the questionnaire. It may be that the rapid acceptance of the total communication philosophy tended to place initial emphasis on the manual aspect with some apparent deterioration of oral skills in a number of programs. However, I believe that this is understandable, since the manual communication element was relatively new to many in the profession and there was a need to develop teacher competencies in this area. As instructors become proficient, I think we will see a refocus on a balanced approach to both modes. I would suggest, further, that total communication programs reinforce the aural/oral program by scheduling separate class periods and individual therapy in auditory training, lipreading, and speech. With this kind of planning, I foresee a continued flourishing of the philosophy in the future. Studies in dissemination have shown that innovations with a high rate of adoption tend to have a low rate of discontinuance, and, indeed, a high degree of integration into the life styles of the receivers (19).

Deaf children do become deaf adults and they need to adjust and to be comfortable in situations involving both the deaf and the hearing. It remains vitally important to provide optimum emphasis for each component of the philosophy so that both modes are enhanced and become mutually supportive.

14

E. Ross Stuckless, Ph.D.

Manual and Graphic Communication

Dr. Stuckless is director of the Office for Integrative Research, at the National Technical Institute for the Deaf, Rochester, New York.

A basic definition of communication, and one that reflects the direction of this article, might be stated as "the transmission of a message from one person to another." By the same token, "effective" communication occurs to the extent that the perception of the message by the receiver matches the intent of the sender.

Effective communication has several prerequisites, each of which can be illustrated relative to manual and to graphic communication.* First, both the sender and receiver must know the *code* in which the message is being transmitted. The code might be English, Sign, or the common understanding that red may mean stop or danger. Second, the *medium* selected for the transmission of the message must be compatible with the abilities of the sender and receiver to use that medium. A deaf adult, for example, may know the English code, but he or she must also have the speech intelligibility necessary for transmitting a message in an oral/aural medium if that is chosen. Similarly, a deaf child must have handwriting or typing skills in order to transmit a message in a graphic medium. Relative to the language of signs, knowledge of a sign vocabulary does not in itself assure the ability to send and receive effectively in that medium. Third, the effectiveness of the medium varies with the *purpose* of the message. This is simply to say that no single medium of communication is equally appropriate for all communicative purposes, even though the first two prerequisites may be met. For example, speaking and/or signing may be effective for conversational purposes, and print (e.g., the textbook) for the storage and retrieval of information. Finally, the effectiveness of the communication medium varies with *external factors*. Both lipreading and manual communication require a direct line of sight between the sender and receiver, and reasonable lighting. Some media require equipment. In order for two deaf people to communicate graphically via teletypewriter, for example, they must each have a TTY in good working order.

---

*For the purposes of this article, manual is defined as the language of signs and its variations, together with fingerspelling; graphic is defined as the representation of English in written and printed form, including text, captions, and electronic displays of English.

The focus of this article is on manual and on graphic communication as media of communication with and among deaf people. This is not to discount speaking, listening, and speechreading as important components in the communication repertoire of the deaf person.

Manual Communication

There is a recent but growing body of research literature on manual communication, particularly as it relates to the deaf child. Much of this literature has been reviewed elsewhere (11, 18, 12). Most of these studies have been designed to study the effects of manual communication upon other aspects of the development of the deaf student, such as English, speech intelligibility, and social development. While Nix (12), and usually the investigators themselves, have been critical of the designs and conclusiveness of each of these studies, the collective weight of the findings is generally supportive of introducing young deaf children to manual communication.

Unfortunately, most of the early studies were conducted on an "ex post facto" rather than longitudinal basis, and selected deaf children of signing deaf parents for comparison with deaf children of hearing parents. Several valid reservations have been expressed about this group of studies. First, none drew comparisons between deaf children with manual communication and deaf children in a home setting highly conducive to oral language development. In a recent effort to shed light on this question, Brasel and Quigley (3) examined the relative performance of four groups of deaf students, including one "intensive oral" group, on a number of measures of English proficiency. Performance consistently favored the "manual English" or signed English group over the other three groups, which also included an "average manual" and "average oral" group, leading the investigators to conclude that while some general advantage may be present in early manual communication for the development of English skills, "greatest advantage appears to come when the parents are competent in standard English and use manual English with and around the child (p. 133)." It should be noted that Brasel and Quigley did not extend their study to an examination of speech intelligibility or lipreading skills among their four groups.

Another question asked about this group of studies is whether the superior performance of the deaf children of deaf parents could be directly attributed to early manual communication or whether some other factors, such as parental acceptance associated with the deaf parents, was responsible. Corson (4) recently compared the performance of a small group of deaf students at The Clarke School for the Deaf whose parents were both oral and deaf, with a group of peers at the same school whose parents were hearing. His findings indicated significantly superior performance on the part of the deaf students of oral deaf parents in reading, arithmetic, and speechreading. He also found that the deaf parents of deaf children expressed more positive acceptance toward deafness than did the hearing parents of deaf children. It should be noted that in studying two additional parallel groups of students at the American School for the Deaf, one of which had signing deaf parents, he encountered similar findings.

In the judgment of the author, the research literature provides a tenable rationale for introducing young deaf children to a sign system; however, many questions remain.

There is mounting evidence that deaf children, under amenable conditions, can develop a sign code on approximately the same developmental timetable as hearing children in developing an English code (1). Numerous investigators have or are in the process of describing how the American Sign Language Code develops among deaf children with deaf parents (6), and how Signed English develops among deaf children with hearing parents who use that code (5).

Signed English probably has greater appeal among hearing parents than American Sign Language because it relates to an English code which the parent already possesses, and because it may enable the child to acquire conventional English skills more readily (3, 2). There is a need for longitudinal research to examine more thoroughly the transfer effects of a sign code into an English code.

Relative to the definition of communication and the several prerequisites for effective communication suggested earlier, it has already been indicated that interest in the study of the code of the language of signs is increasing. However, there is relatively little current research activity on the effectiveness of manual communication as a medium for information transmission, and even less on the communication purposes to which it is particularly well or poorly suited. Given that two persons have a common manual code, are their manual and visual-perceptual abilities to send and receive the message adequate? For example, most hearing learners-of-signs observe that they develop the ability to send a signed message before they learn to receive it. When does the deaf child develop the visual skills necessary for decoding fingerspelling and Signed English? These and many related questions seek answers.

There has been some exploratory work on the "intactness" of a message when it is communicated manually. Hoemann and Tweney (10) presented some English text material to native signers, asking them to translate the material into signs which were videotaped. A second group of native signers observed the videotaped signed material and was asked to translate this material without having seen the original English text. When the original English and the back translation were compared, they were found to be very close. This presupposed that the participants in the experiment possessed both an English and a sign code. In another study, Hoemann (9) asked several pairs of hearing and deaf children to use spoken English and manual communication, respectively, to complete three tasks that required communication. Performance of the hearing pairs was significantly better than that of the deaf pairs, but Hoemann attributed this more to an experiential deficit on the part of the deaf children than to the communication medium itself. One might ask, however, whether each member of each deaf pair had the manual code necessary for the communication. Also, one might infer that, in this instance, a manual medium was not appropriate to the purpose of the tasks.

Indeed, the effectiveness of a medium of communication cannot be detached from the purpose for which it is intended. The author once asked his deaf brother why he sometimes speaks and sometimes communicates with strangers by note. The response was that, if a waiter brought him the wrong vegetable, that was tolerable, but a valve job instead of an oil change was not. Unfortunately, some people, hearing and deaf, tend to attach a positive or negative valence to manual communication without due attention to the purpose for which it is being used. In the author's judgment, it is imperative that we begin to address ourselves more openly to those communication conditions among deaf children that lend themselves to manual communication and those that do not. To further complicate the problem, we must take into account the other prerequisites of effective communication, complementary and alternative media, and most important, the aptitudes and educational goals of the individual child. Weiss, Goodwin, and Moores (19) in a longitudinal study of the interactions among the characteristics of young deaf children and variables associated with early intervention programs are endeavoring to come to grips with some of the myriad variables involved.

Before turning to graphic communication, brief mention should be made of external factors influencing the effectiveness of manual communication as a medium. We know remarkably little, for example, about such variables as optimum distance and horizontal angle between the sender and receiver, lighting, and background. These kinds of questions may have particular importance for groups of deaf people in interacting with one another or following an interpreter.

A society ultimately determines the languages and communication media it will use. In this regard, more specialists, and particularly linguists and psycholinguists, are becoming absorbed in studying sign as a language. The working vocabulary of the language of signs is increasing. Increasing numbers of hearing people are learning to communicate manually, to the extent that it has been estimated that more hearing people now know the language of signs than do deaf people. As more people learn the code and how to use it, its usefulness to deaf people as a medium within their communication repertoire should increase correspondingly.

Graphic Communication

The development of English language skills among deaf students is given high priority by parents and teachers, as should be. Knowledge of the English code is essential to effective oral communication, (i.e. speaking, listening, and lipreading) and to graphic communication (i.e., reading and writing).

There is a considerable body of anecdotal and research literature on the English language development of deaf students, for the most part focusing on: a) strategies for enabling the child to acquire the English code, such as approaches to teaching the structure of English, and b) assessment of the level of mastery of the code, such as estimates of reading achievement. In 1966 several excellent reviews of some of this literature were brought together in a special publication of *The Volta Review* (16).

In this chapter's section on manual communication, it was observed that increasing attention is being given to the process whereby a deaf child develops a sign code. Parallel activity has also centered on how deaf children develop an English code, particularly as expressed through writing. Noteworthy, both for the findings it presents and for its excellent review of the related literature, is a recently completed report of a study of the syntactic structures in the language of deaf children by Quigley, Wilbur, Power, Montanelli, and Steinkamp (17). In their report of this study, conducted with representative 10- to 18-year-old deaf students nationally, the authors conclude that the structure of language expressed through writing by deaf students is essentially similar in kind to that used by hearing students who are greatly retarded developmentally.

Presumably, this developmental lag in the mastery of the English code persists into adulthood. Hammermeister (8), in the only study known to the author that has addressed itself to this question, found little change in the reading performance of deaf adults several years after they had graduated from high school.

Up to this point we have been discussing various aspects of shaping and describing the English code in deaf children, and not functional applications of English to reading and writing for communication. The author has often noted a tendency on the part of teachers to say, "We communicate orally," or "We use total communication." Teachers are much less likely to say, "We communicate graphically," in spite of their frequent use of the chalkboard, slot charts, ditto sheets, books, the overhead projector, and captioned films. While graphic communication is used extensively in most classrooms for the purpose of transmitting messages to and from the student, particularly those beyond the earliest grade levels, there is a tendency to regard reading and writing more as skills to be learned than as a medium to be used for communication at the time.

This brings us to the question of the abilities of the sender and receiver to use a graphic medium, given that they have an English code. Both speaking and writing require an English code. However, assuming that the child has the necessary motor abilities, it is without doubt much easier for a child to master handwriting or typing skills than articulation and intelligible speech. By the same token, the visual-perceptual skills (as separate from the English code) involved in reading print are probably more readily acquired than those involved in the deaf child's learning to use his residual hearing and to speechread. Print is spatial, while voice transmission is temporal and not as conducive to processing through vision.

A series of experiments conducted with postsecondary deaf students at the National Technical Institute for the Deaf (7, 14) and with secondary-level students (14, 20) have reported better reception of verbal information by students when this information was presented graphically, (i.e., print and/or videotaped captions) than when the same information was presented manually or orally. It should be added that none of the oral presentations were made under ideal conditions. Additionally, students were required to respond to typed questions as the response mode, which may have favored the groups receiving the graphically-presented material.

Norwood (13) tested the ability of college-educated and noncollege-educated deaf adults to process information presented on a nationally televised news broadcast when captions and an interpreter were added. Results were favorable to the captioned presentation for both groups and particularly among the college-educated viewers.

It would be erroneous to conclude from these studies that graphic communication is categorically superior to other communication media for deaf people who possess an English code. One must examine each medium relative to its purpose. At this time graphic communication does not lend itself well to real-time, interactive communication, whereas oral and manual media do.

Early in this chapter, it was suggested that the effectiveness of a communication medium is related to external factors. One can view the status and applications of technology as a factor external to, but impinging on, communication. This is well illustrated by the development of the hearing aid. We can look to technology to give great assistance in establishing graphic communication as a more useful medium for deaf people in the future. Several notable accomplishments have already taken place. We have had captioned films for some time, both for educational and entertainment purposes. Numerous nationally produced television programs are now being captioned for deaf viewers.

Although it was suggested earlier that graphic communication is not conducive to real-time verbal interaction, this is not strictly so. The teletypewriter and other telecommunication devices with electronic graphic displays now permit deaf people to interact at distances in ways not possible a few years ago.

Of enormous promise, both in helping deaf children establish the English code visually and for making graphic communication truly real-time, is the technological potential for automatic speech recognition. With the aid of computer technology and speech science, it should become both feasible and widely practical for a person's speech to be automatically transposed into graphics, allowing the deaf child and adult literally to read the voice. This should enable graphic communication to become a more versatile medium and greatly accelerate the child's mastery of the English code.

A number of broad research needs have been implicitly or explicitly suggested in this article. There is a pressing need to give more attention to the applications of language to communication while maintaining our attention on the language developmental process. Communication is inclusive of, but not synonomous with, language.

The deaf child has a complex set of tasks. He or she must not only acquire the available codes but must also learn how to apply these codes appropriately and selectively in a variety of media. Both as parents and educators, and as cocommunicators with the child, so must we. ⚏

15   *Frank B. Withrow, Ph.D.*

Applications of Technology to Communication

Dr. Withrow is special assistant to the deputy commissioner, Bureau of Education for the Handicapped, Office of Education, United States Department of Health, Education, and Welfare.

Scientists and educators who have worked with the hearing impaired for a number of years have felt that a breakthrough might be possible through the development of technological aids for the deaf. Without negating the benefits that have been achieved by the developments to date, it is fair to say that no aid has been so dramatic that it offers the hearing impaired person an alternative system that fully compensates for his or her loss of hearing. All aids require a long period of training in their use before they reach their maximum benefit to the user.

Aids may be classified as two distinct types: a) sensory aids, which either amplify the signal for the deficient sensory system or transform the stimuli so that it can be used by an alternate sensory system and b) educational aids, which may or may not be specifically designed for the hearing impaired population. The sensory aid attempts to either by-pass or override the deficient sensory system. On the other hand the educational aid tends to store and retrieve knowledge for the learner in formats such as textbooks, computer assisted instruction, or programmed instruction.

Sensory Aids

The learner gains knowledge and skills through sensory experiences that are coded into symbolic form that may be shared with other learners. In the normal development of a child, his distance senses (sight and sound) rapidly become his major contact with his environment. Until the infant achieves a degree of mobility, touch and taste also play an important role in his sensory awareness and exploration of the world about him. As adults we have learned to code these sensory stimuli into symbols that are used in communicating our thoughts and experiences.

102

To understand the possible uses of technology for the hearing impaired, it is important to understand the characteristics of vision, audition, and touch; because it is most likely that the child will learn to organize his world and develop his symbol system through these sense organs. Helmholtz (5) pointed out that the eye's ". . . extraordinary value depends upon the way in which we use it; its perfection is practical, not absolute, consisting not in the avoidance of every error, but in the fact that all its defects do not prevent its rendering us the most important and varied services." Geldard (4) expanded upon these observations by summarizing them into a single statement that "the eye is the great perceiver of spatial relations; it is beautifully adapted to the world of space." Geldard further elaborates and discusses Helmholtz's understanding of the function of the ear. Helmholtz (6) noted that "the ear is eminently the organ for small intervals of time."

Geldard (4), in summarizing the receptive channels that can deal with time and space, brings to our attention the fact that "the sense of touch, (is) the only remaining receptive channel in the body having any solid claim to substantial discriminatory powers where either space or time is concerned. The skin does well, very well, with time, far surpassing the eye in this respect and even rivaling the ear in some circumstances. It also far outstrips audition as a spatial sense but, in this regard, clearly has to knuckle under to vision."

Scientists have come a long way in their search for an external ear for the hearing impaired child, but they remain short of their anticipated goal. We know that any device that has promise of working will need to have several characteristics. One of the most significant characteristics will be a long period of training in the use of the device. We have enough information on the various sensory systems to know that the substituted sensory system should have some of the same characteristics as the original sensory system. The sense of touch transmits temporal stimuli in ways very much like the sense of hearing. The sense of vision can display, or have displayed for it, temporal stimuli in spatial signals. Obviously, print is a spatial array of the spoken word.

The characteristics of an aid that will be most meaningful to the hearing impaired child are as follows:

- It must have the capacity to pick up auditory symbols (spoken words) from any direction.
- It must transform the auditory code to a substituted sensory code on a temporal and real-time basis.
- It must be compatible with the residual hearing of the user, so that there is a synergestic relation between the new stimuli and the traditional stimuli.
- It must be reliable, portable, and cosmetically suitable for the user, so that it does not interfere with the normal life functions of the user.

Sherrick (8) has termed these prosthetic devices as metastatic aids, that is, aids that transform sensory signals meant for one sensory system into stimuli that can be detected and used by another sensory system. To a degree we have always done this with hearing impaired people. The use of the language of signs and lipreading are, in effect, metastatic systems designed to have the eye take over for the ear. There is a long history of experiments that have sought to use the skin to receive spoken stimuli and the eye to transpose spoken stimuli. Gault and Crane (3) explored the use of vibrations to the skin to transmit spoken information. Their efforts were crude but significant, because they were able to demonstrate some success in enabling persons to discriminate sound from stimulation of the skin. Work in this area has slowly progressed and today there are a number of tactual vocoders that have been used in basic experimentation in training deaf youngsters. Engelmann and Rosov (2) have developed a tactual vocoder with which one deaf subject learned to discriminate 150 words in a 48-week period. Some of the conclusions of these investigators are that: "Deaf subjects can be taught to hear fine speech discriminations through the tactual mode, even discriminations as fine as those involved in *fly . . . . sly* or *teef . . . . teeth*."

They go on to say that "the tactual experiment provides a unique glimpse into the amount and type of practice needed for a person to learn to use a new sensory modality. The performance of these deaf children is encouraging. With more sophisticated and portable hardware, we believe that a deaf infant could learn to hear, using tactual input in exactly the same way a hearing child learns to hear."

Other investigators (7) have demonstrated the use of a vocoder belt which is worn around the abdomen. This system uses 20 channels or stimulators whose filter-center frequencies were preset at approximately 1/3 octave intervals. The frequency range covers 190 to 6200 Hz. To date, several studies have been conducted with this system using both hearing and deaf subjects. Subjects have been able to discriminate vowel placement, voiced and voiceless consonants, and nasalization. Subjects who have been trained under the McGinnis Association Method have been able to distinguish connected dialogue using only the vocoder.

Work has also been done with research into the use of vision as the substitute mode for speech reception. A number of studies have tried to develop visible speech. Some of the more current and promising of these systems are those which use visual information to supplement lipreading. The Upton (10) glasses are an example of this type of aid. These glasses provide clues as to voiced/voiceless, stops and fricatives through the use of dots of lights in the glasses. Experimentation with these materials has shown that people can learn to lipread with greater proficiency using these aids.

Visible speech has been pursued by a number of investigators for many years. Many of these attempts have used sophisticated electronic analyzers, and others have devised human systems such as cued speech (1). All of these systems have to a degree been able to demonstrate some improvement in some aspects of communication or signal detection. Many of the tests of these systems have used syllable or word recognition tasks that do not indicate the effectiveness of the system in connected speech.

Educational Aids

Educational aids have always played an important role in the education of the hearing impaired child. Early teachers used pictures, models, and pantomime to help the young hearing impaired child build his or her knowledge of the world. Early speech teachers working with the hearing impaired used diagrams of the tongue, teeth, and lips as well as hand signals to depict the position of the articulators in speech. Many prominent educators of the hearing impaired felt that the development of the motion picture would revolutionize the education of hearing impaired people. Max Goldstein, the founder of Central Institute for the Deaf, created a small operational museum for use by his pupils. This museum included such things as industrial exhibits, natural exhibits, and a wide range of stereoptican slides that were used as learning resources for pupils attending the institute.

John A. Gough, the first director of Captioned Films for the Deaf, pointed out that the introduction of the "talking motion picture" was a temporary setback for hearing impaired people. The old silent, subtitled motion pictures were unique in that they were a technology that equalized the deaf and hearing audiences. For a short time the hearing audience was "deafened" when they went to a motion picture and the gap between the hearing impaired and the hearing person was narrowed. Consequently, when the sound motion picture was developed the differences between the deaf and hearing audiences were broadened. Sound motion pictures and eventually television increased the available information that is accessible to the hearing world. It was not until 1958 when the U. S. Congress passed Public Law 85-905. (Captioned Films for the Deaf Act) that deaf people had partial access to the avalanche of entertainment, news, and educational materials made available by the technology of mass communications.

Stepp (9) has developed a language learning laboratory for the hard of hearing child. He utilized the principles that had been developed for hearing children learning a foreign language and tape machines, and adapted these principles for use with 8mm cartridge film loops. These loops carry visual and auditory information and are designed to cycle so that, when one pupil has completed his work, the teaching booth is ready for the next learner. The manipulative kits are nonverbal and the film teacher always instructs the pupil to return the kit to its proper place as the lesson is finished.

Withrow (11), under a contract with Captioned Films for the Deaf, has developed a series of language development films that use silent 8mm loops for lipreading and the language master for auditory training. Withrow and Stepp have combined their efforts and produced a series of noun vocabulary films that have been released for use in a number of schools for the deaf throughout the nation. These films are so cued that there are stimulus and response signals enabling the pupil to use the films without completely recycling the film loop. The pupil can use a flash card as a response set or respond by writing the correct response.

Perhaps the most significant development of the late 1960's and early 1970's has been the establishment of the regional media centers for the deaf. These centers provide a basis for training of personnel in the use of media with hearing impaired learners. Marshall Hester developed the Southwestern Regional Media Center for the Deaf in New Mexico in 1964, Robert Stepp developed the Midwestern Regional Media Center for the Deaf in 1965, William Jackson established the Southeastern Regional Media Center for the Deaf in 1966, and Raymond Wyman developed the Northeastern Regional Media Center for the Deaf in 1966. Each one of these centers specializes in a given area of media. Hester and Wyman greatly contributed to the use of the overhead projector in schools and classes for the deaf. Jackson specialized in television and captioning of television. Stepp provided leadership in the development of motion picture film for use in schools and classes for the deaf. He also established an annual symposium on the use of technology in the education of the deaf, bringing together educators, technologists, and decision-makers in schools and classes for the deaf. The symposium has provided a theoretical model for the use and implementation of a learning technology as applied to the hearing impaired learner.

A major objective of the Captioned Films for the Deaf Branch, under the leadership of John A. Gough and later Gilbert Delgado, has been to provide a minimum base of technological equipment for every classroom serving deaf youngsters throughout the land. This means that each classroom must be provided with a screen, an overhead projector, and a filmstrip projector. The implementation of this longrange goal began in the mid-1960's and was essentially completed in the later 1960's. The unique concept of the federal government loaning both equipment and materials to schools and classes for the deaf developed an acceptance of the use of technology as a major part of their learning system within the administrative structures of many schools and programs for the deaf and hard of hearing. As money began to become available through other federal funds, such as Public Law 89-313 and Part B of the Education of the Handicapped Act (EHA), local and state education agencies began to adopt their own systems of technology, which included computer assisted instruction and closed circuit television. The federal role has remained one of providing "courseware" in the forms of films and television programs.

Schools for the deaf have installed comprehensive television systems that allow for a wide range of use of this medium. Many schools have their own capability to caption programs that they have videotaped off the air. Others have various television capabilities producing a wide range of local or in-school programs. Still other systems have limited their production capabilities to "portapacks," which provide the teacher and pupil a tool for use on field trips or other activities outside the classroom.

Several major curriculum projects have been funded over the years by the media branches of the U. S. Bureau of Education for the Handicapped. The most long term project has been Language Instruction to Facilitate Education (Project LIFE), which ran for 13 years and required a $3,2000,000 capitalization. It is currently being distributed through a commercial concern to a wide market of handicapped and nonhandicapped learners. The federal government receives a royalty from the sales of these materials. Other materials have also been developed and distributed either in the loan and distribution system of the Bureau or through the commercial market. Massive distribution of materials such as those developed by Project LIFE can be effectively distributed through the normal marketing processes.

The hearing impaired person has been at a disadvantage in the vital area of news and information. Under the leadership of Malcolm J. Norwood, Chief, Captioned Films and Telecommunications Branch, Bureau of Education for the Handicapped, U.S. Office of Education, new breakthroughs have emerged in the field of captioned television. The two types of captioned television currently being aired are closed captions and open captions. Closed captions are a special system which broadcasts a coded signal requiring a decoder to make them visible. The decoder can be attached to a personal TV set or to a local broadcast or cable television station. It transmits the captions in a form visible on a TV receiver (open captions). Open captions are those which are visible at the normal broadcast time of the program. For example, the ABC Evening News is captioned in open captions by WGBH, Boston, and then rebroadcast across the nation at a later time. Currently, there are between two to four hours of new captioned programming that enter the system each week. The Adams Chronicles, for example, is being captioned. The Public Broadcasting Service (PBS) provides these materials in closed captioned formats on the nights of their normal broadcast and in open captions during the second broadcast. More than three-quarters of the PBS stations across the nation carry some form of captioned television.

The next step in the advancement of the use of technology with the hearing impaired may come in the blending of the sensory aid and the educational aid into a single system. The output of a computer-assisted instructional program may be paired with a sensory interface, which can provide the hearing impaired learner signals partially replacing those he cannot detect because of his hearing loss. A systematic use of such a system may provide the foundations required for the hearing impaired child to learn language and other fundamental concepts required in a basic education.

16 Philip A. Bellefleur, Ph.D.

TTY Communication: Its History and Future

Dr. Bellefleur is headmaster of The Pennsylvania School for the Deaf, Philadelphia.

Telecommunications for the Deaf, or TTY as it is abbreviated, is a system of transmitting the word-characters from one geographic location to another. Two teleprinters are electronically linked together transmitting on a standard telephone line. When a word is typed at one end of the line, it is transmitted via telephone as a tone-code to the other teleprinter where it is reconverted into word form, thus allowing deaf persons to communicate with hearing individuals or other deaf. This simple communications concept is probably the most exciting happening for the deaf since the invention of the hearing aid at the turn of the century.

In a sense, when Alexander Graham Bell developed the telephone, he inadvertently set the progress of the deaf backward by almost a century. The invention of the phone advanced the potential of hearing people an untold amount by allowing them to communicate over distances at nearly the speed of light. While hearing persons were sharing ideas and meeting new friends around the globe, the deaf remained much the same as always, restricted in their communication by the distance they could see, the time it took to mail and receive a letter, or the drive across town to speak to a friend. The relative communication differential between the deaf and the hearing person continued to widen as telephony continued to grow.

This ever expanding differential should have ended in 1964 when Robert Weitbrecht, a profoundly deaf American physicist, successfully developed an acoustic/inductive coupler allowing two teletype machines to communicate with each other over a standard telephone line. One would think that the deaf would have literally beaten a path to Dr. Weitbrecht's door, but in the four years between 1964 and 1968, only 25 TTY's were operational. Between April 1968 and June 1975, there was a meteoric rise of machines registered with the official Teletype Association for the Deaf,* but considering that the total during this period was less than 5,000 units, it

---

* writers for the Deaf, Inc. (T.D.I.)
x 28332, Washington, D.C. 20013

is obvious that, at the present rate of growth, it will take many years to provide each household with a teleprinter. More startling is the knowledge that, of the TTY's now registered to be in operation, most Model 15's and 19's are machines designed by the Teletype Corporation 40 to 45 years ago.

Despite obvious growth problems, TTY is exploding the communication potential of the average deaf person. He need no longer be restricted, inconvenienced, and even endangered by his limited hearing. Telecommunications is an electronic ear/voice that literally projects him receptively and expressively around the world.

Telecommunications is bringing to the deaf the same joys and sorrows that telephony brought to the hearing person about a century ago. It is a system that carries responsibilities as well as privileges, and punishments as well as rewards. Already there are countless stories of life and death taking place on the teleprinter. A prowler is apprehended because someone owned a TTY and cared enough to notify the police; the home of a hearing person is saved because a deaf neighbor could "call" the Fire Department. As the deaf person is caught up in the momentum of telecommunications, teen-age children are being asked to stop tying up the TTY machine; husbands are calling wives to say they will be working late. The obscene TTY call has already happened and the TTY solicitor of magazine subscriptions is surely close behind.

Present Status of TTY

Curiously, the present system, using the behemoth-like Model 15's and 19's, is growing. And yet, with more than 10 years of development, the system is not much different from the original concept developed by Weitbrecht in 1964. In spite of the interest by a half-dozen electronic manufacturers, in spite of expressed interest from governmental agencies in the United States, and in spite of legislation introduced into the United States Congress, little has been done to put a modern electronic TTY terminal in the hands of the average deaf person at a price he or she can afford.

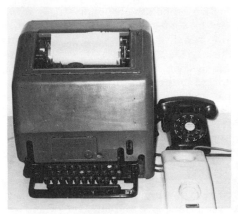

TTY Model 15. Photo courtesy of the Teletype Corporation.

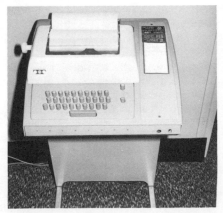

TTY Model 32. Photo courtesy of the Teletype Corporation.

Perhaps in his wisdom Dr. Weitbrecht anticipated this lack of support, for it would seem as though he purposely designed the TTY around out-of-date but freely available equipment. But whether by design or accident, this fact has been responsible for keeping the entire system alive and even expanding.

The modern equivalent of the Model 15 is the Model 32 hard-copy teleprinter. Like the older units, the "32" produces paper copy at speeds of up to 60 words per minute.

Although more attractive than its predecessors, the "32" is still too large for home use, and its $800 price is prohibitive. An interesting aspect of "hard" copy, or paper copy, is that hearing impaired people have come to feel that a written record is a must. Apparently, having the printed words in hand allows the individual to reread and study the communication at his leisure. It can also be used for record keeping or showing to other members of the family at a later time. Unfortunately, paper copy machines are heavy and costly. Even now it is possible to use a tape recorder to reproduce the TTY code for later replay but, as yet, this method has not proven itself particularly popular with the deaf as a substitute for an immediate paper copy.

In fairness, several manufacturers have attempted to design modern equipment, and three of these presently sell instruments in the United States. Again, the price is from $600 to $1200, depending on the unit and the options selected. This is obviously prohibitive for the average deaf individual with a median personal income of $5,915 per year (1). If the newborn TTY industry is unable to grow, or worse, if it begins to fail because of economic limitations of the deaf, the solution may rest with temporary support by the federal government.

The design of the new TTY equipment has taken one of two forms. For lack of available terms, I call one an "electronic word-scan" and the other a "TV word machine." The device most often seen is the electronic word-scan machine.

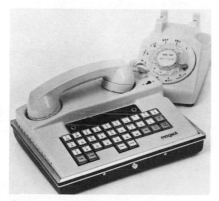

Photo courtesy of Magsat Corporation.

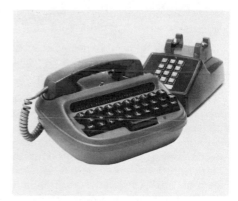

Photo courtesy of Micon Industries.

Scan machines operate on essentially the same principle as the old TTY units. One dials the number on a standard telephone, places the phone on a coupler, and types out words on a modified typewriter keyboard. A flashing light on the unit informs the caller whether the line is free or busy. APCOM Corporation of California has a system that even answers the phone automatically and informs the caller about how to leave a message. Unlike teletype machines that produce words on paper, word-scan devices form the letter character on a display unit similar to the displays in electronic calculators. As one types, words begin to move across the scanner in much the same manner as the electronic news broadcast at Times Square in New York City. Most word scanners have a line containing 32 characters or less. As one looks at the unit, words seem to appear on the right, move along for a while, and finally disappear on the left.

The second device, the television-word machine, is actually a modified cathode ray tube (CRT) terminal, similar to the devices used in airports to schedule flights.

Television-word machines produce only written words on a television screen; they do not produce any type of picture image. Words appear on the lower right of the TV screen and proceed along in much the same manner as the electronic word-scan machine. However, when a line is completed, it moves upward on the screen, remaining visible to the sender and receiver. This process is repeated until the screen is filled with sentences.

Finally, the sentences at the top disappear, one by one, as new text comes into view at the bottom.

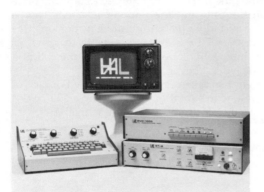
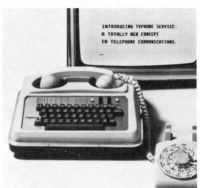

Photo courtesy of HAL Communications Corporation.   Photo courtesy of Phonics Corporation.

The subject of television-picture-phones is sufficiently important to devote some space to its history. Unlike the television-word machine described earlier, it is a true picture-producing device. The system has a camera, a miniature TV set, and a telephone hand-set, all built into the same unit. At least two companies have been experimenting with television-picture-phones; one is the Stromberg-Carlson Corporation and the other is Bell Telephone Laboratories, a subsidiary of Western Electronic and American Telephone and Telegraph Company. Neither instrument was designed with the needs of the hearing impaired in mind. Moreover, most engineers agree that the picture telephone as a residential consumer item is at least 15 and probably 20 years away. The Bell Company is experimenting with three systems presently, but the only operational unit for the deaf is a Stromberg-Carlson intercommunications system at the National Technical Institute for the Deaf. All are unsuitable, in their present form, for widespread public use.

TTY Extended Services

In addition to interpersonal communications, such as two hearing impaired people, or a hearing impaired and a hearing person communicating via the TTY, there is the entire concept of TTY services.

Some large cities in the United States, for example, now provide one of two types of emergency links with the deaf community. The first of these is an indirect connection with a message agency that usually maintains a 24-hour TTY monitoring system to relay calls for police, fire, or ambulance. In the second type, available in a few areas of the country, a direct TTY call is possible with the police or fire department, who maintain a teleprinter especially for the deaf community.

Since the relay-message service is a service in itself, it deserves some discussion here. Though variations exist, the deaf person usually dials a special number and his/her call is received by a hearing volunteer using a TTY. A voice call is then made to the person or agency that the deaf person wishes to contact. The volunteer conveys the information and returns same. Conversely, if a hearing person wishes to communicate with a deaf person, the process is reversed. Most message agencies restrict callers to business or emergency use, but a few will handle social calls. The service varies from place to place; some message services are free, while others charge. One of the largest organizations serving the deaf in this way is CONTACT, an agency of the United Methodist Church. CONTACT is an international telephone "help" service aiding the elderly, the infirmed, and the troubled. In some areas, this organization has also volunteered to provide a voice link for the deaf by maintaining a 24-hour TTY service.

In a few cities, the deaf are beginning to enjoy the privilege of catalogue shopping. Sears & Roebuck and John Wanamaker, in Philadelphia, maintain a TTY service. Shopping in this way is not for the meek. Mistakes are quite common, and it takes a fair amount of patience and good language to purchase things by teleprinter.

Public pay-telephone-teletype services are also available. At The Pennsylvania School for the Deaf, and Lexington School for the Deaf, for example, persons may make unassisted local calls. The system works much the same as the home TTY except for the necessity of putting money into the phone. Long distance calls pose more of a problem and require the help of a hearing person to interact with the telephone operator. Little success has been made in convincing telephone companies to install TTY's in their offices, but this, of course, is the only solution to the unassisted long distance pay-telephone service to the deaf.

Amtrak, the National Railroad Passenger Corporation, is the newest service addition to the teletype network. It is now possible to get information on Amtrak buses and trains by dialing 1-800-523-6590 (in Philadelphia the number is 1-800-562-6960).

Throughout the United States, cities such as Philadelphia, Washington, New York, and St. Louis maintain "news centers" for the deaf. They are referred to as "hardwire" or "telephone news centers" because, to receive news, the individual must dial a special number and wait for the news to print out on his or her TTY machine. Most news operations in the United States are of this type. Their principle disadvantage is their inability to give news to more than one person at a time. Since most teleprinters can only copy 60 words per minute, even a short message can tie up the line for a long time. A limited number of news centers use tape recorders and can handle several callers at one time, but magnetic tape does not reproduce the TTY tones well, especially over the phone, and special digital tape reproductions are beyond the budget of most centers, or subscribers. Most tend to be very limited in scope, serving only the needs and interests of the local citizens.

In the very near future, The Pennsylvania School for the Deaf plans to open the first Radio TTY news station in the United States and, perhaps, the first in the world. Sponsored by a grant from a private foundation, the news center will broadcast to a projected TTY population of 1,000 families of the hearing impaired in five countries. Initially, the broadcast will last for two hours and be repeated three times a day. As the experimental station matures, its broadcast will increase in length. The content of the news will be local, national, and international, with news of the school and hearing impaired community as well. A unique feature of the center will be the use of hearing impaired youth as editorial staff. Honor students will be selected to rewrite United Press International and other news into language that can be better understood by the average deaf person.

Technically speaking, Radio TTY consists of sending taped TTY codes to a transmitter where they are mixed with a high-frequency carrier wave and beamed out to the deaf community. Each recipient will have a small radio tuner that excludes the carrier signal and leaves the TTY signal code. In audible form again, the signals trigger the TTY machine and are reconverted back into written words.

News centers have several hidden benefits to the hearing impaired community—stimulation of personal growth, stimulation of community growth, and self-perpetuation of the TTY network itself.

Finally, one of the earliest efforts in supportive services is the "Blue Book." This small, hardcover, loose-leaf book contains an alphabetical and zip code listing of most of the TTY stations in the United States. It is published by the Teletypewriters for the Deaf, Inc., and is free to individuals who are members of T.D.I. Listings in the directory are also free.

Often I am asked, "What is the future of telecommunications for the deaf?" A better question would be, "What will its impact be on the growth of the deaf community?" In answer to the first question, humanity's progress in technology is in direct proportion to the tools at its disposal. When there was only a hammer, people could only pound on things; when the knife was developed they began to cut; and when the telephone was invented, they began to communicate by wire over long distances. The future of telecommunications includes, in order of probable appearance:

• Miniaturized, all electronic TTY machines with built-in CRT-like screens;

• TTY with computer capability for interfacing with educational computer systems;

• Captioned TV programs on a regular basis, visible only to the deaf;

• TV phone with picture and word capability. The early models will be designed for hearing people with later models modified for the deaf;

• Symbol converting typewriters that convert speech to the printed word and the printed word into speech, allowing all hearing and deaf persons to communicate directly.

Obviously, the future also holds concepts such as a "time operator," "weather operator," "dial-a-prayer," or "dial-a-poem," and other bourgeois services available to most people now. But the future of communications for the deaf will be more than machines and more than dial-a-prayer services.

The TTY will have a total impact on the growth of a community that has been unparalleled since the invention of the hearing aid at the turn of the century. A network of communication will develop that brings together a mini-society within the larger one and facilitates an exchange of information between the members of both groups. It will motivate deaf students and stimulate achievement—but most of all, it will bring deaf and hearing persons closer together.

17

Samuel F. Lybarger

Personal Hearing Aids

Mr. Lybarger, an acoustical consultant, was formerly president of Radioear Corporation.

The development of personal electrical hearing aids began shortly after the invention of the telephone by Alexander Graham Bell. In this bicentennial year of 1976, we can sample some of the progress made since that time by reviewing a few of the improvements that have taken place during the past decade.

In 1965, according to data of the Hearing Aid Industry Conference, Inc., over 352,000 personal hearing aids were sold in the United States. Of these, approximately 17.3% were conventional or body aids, 29.5% eyeglass aids, 46.9% behind-the-ear aids, and 6.3% in-the-ear aids. Although there was a considerable range in size and weight, somewhat typical weights were 2 ounces for the body aid, 0.4 ounces for the eyeglass aid, 0.25 ounces for the behind-the-ear aid, and 0.15 ounces for the in-the-ear aid. By 1965, all wearable electronic hearing aids employed transistors, which previously had had a profound effect in reducing hearing aid size and battery cost. The prevailing type of microphone in use then was the balanced armature magnetic microphone, which was constantly being reduced in size. Receivers (i.e., earphones) were mostly monopolar or bipolar units for body aids, or balanced armature magnetic receivers for eyeglass, behind-the-ear, and in-the-ear aids.

The hearing aid was reasonably acceptable a decade ago with respect to performance. Average gain (measured instrumentally) ranged from a typical 25 or 30 dB for in-the-ear aids to 50 dB in eyeglass aids and behind-the-ear aids and to 80 dB in very powerful body aids. Frequency range of eyeglass and behind-the-ear aids was on the order of from 450 to 4500 Hz. In the past 10 years, however, revolutionary developments in hearing aid components have resulted in hearing aids that are smaller, more reliable, and, in many cases, more economical of battery power than ever before.

Amplifiers

In 1965, most hearing aid amplifiers were of the discrete type. Separate resistors, transistors, and capacitors were soldered into position, usually on a printed circuit board with an etched copper wiring pattern. This is still a very good construction.

About 1965, integrated circuit amplifiers (IC) appeared. The IC is a device in which the entire amplifier circuit, including transistors, resistors, and diodes are produced on a tiny silicon chip with suitable leads attached. During the past 10 years, ICs for hearing aid use have undergone many improvements. From the simple ICs of 1965 have come units with push-pull outputs for greater power handling capacity, units with the capability for automatic gain control, units with extra gain for telephone coils, and units with very low battery power consumption.

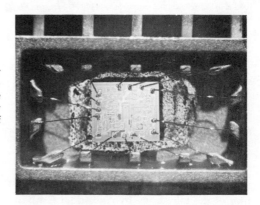

Interior view of an integrated circuit for hearing aid use that includes AGC circuitry. The silicon chip on which the amplifier is produced measures only about .060" by .070". (Photo courtesy of Linear Technology, Inc.)

Parallel improvements have been made via the "hybrid" concept. In these devices, the conductive wiring pattern is printed and fired onto a thin ceramic plate in the thick-film version, or vacuum deposited in the thin-film method. The resistors are deposited onto the plate using various kinds of resistor inks or metals and the necessary transistor chips and capacitors soldered at the appropriate points of the wiring pattern. This type of amplifier is small, rugged, and can be rather easily modified by the manufacturer, should this be desirable.

An important part of the amplifier circuit is the volume control. Recent developments in small volume controls for ear-level aids have made them less susceptible to the effects of perspiration, through the use of neoprene or soft plastic seals and the introduction of a ceramic-metal (cermet) material for the resistance strip. Needless to say, with the diminishing size of hearing aids, volume controls must be small and can be somewhat difficult for some persons to adjust.

One of the important improvements in ear-level aids over the past 10 years has been greater adjustability of such characteristics as gain, saturation output, low frequency response, and degree of compression. This has been made possible by the introduction of tiny rheostats or potentiometers that usually can be set with a small screwdriver. These tiny controls have undergone significant improvement in design during the recent past to obtain greater ruggedness.

The number and quality of hearing aids with automatic gain control has increased markedly in the past few years. Different input-output characteristics of the aids are available. In one form, the output increases linearly as the input is increased up to a "knee" point, above which the output increases slowly or hardly at all. This tends to keep the signal reaching the ear at a fairly constant level for a considerable range of inputs. In another form, the knee point occurs at a low input level and the output increases more rapidly with increasing input, with the objective of complementing the impaired ear's dynamic characteristic. A third form has no sharp knee point, but gradually changes the amount of compression as the intensity increases. Use of compression aids appears to be increasing in the United States.

Microphones

The greatest advances in personal hearing aids since 1965 have been the result of simultaneous performance improvement and size reduction in microphones. To emphasize the reduction in size, Figure 1 the photo below shows a typical 1965 magnetic microphone, a 1975 electret microphone and, for comparison, a familiar coin.

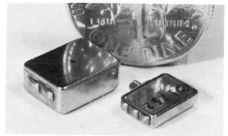

The currently available tiny electret or ceramic microphone at the right is only about one-third as large in volume as the 1965 magnetic microphone at the left. (Units shown were manufactured by Knowles Electronics, Inc.)

The first important development in this period was the introduction of the extremely tiny ceramic microphone for hearing aid use. Ceramic microphones have been in successful use for many years and had been employed in body aids well before 1965. However, they were much too large for ear-level aids. The successful ceramic microphones for small hearing aids were made possible by combining the ceramic microphone element—a thin strip of barium titanate ceramic—with a field-effect transistor and its associated circuitry in a very small metal shielding enclosure. Another important element in the system was the development of precise diaphragms that efficiently convert sound pressure into a vibratory mechanical force to bend the ceramic strip and thus generate a voltage to be amplified.

The basic advantages of the ceramic microphone are its high sensitivity, its wider frequency range (especially in the low frequencies), its flatness of response, and its resistance to mechanical shock and to humidity. Following the ceramic microphone by three or four years, the electret microphone was developed. This is, perhaps, the most important of all developments in the hearing aid field during the past 10 years. The electret microphone uses a self-contained field-effect transistor, as does the ceramic microphone, to give the very high input-impedance needed to utilize the voltage generated by the electret action.

The word "electret" is similar in derivation to the word "magnet" but applies to an electronic instead of a magnetic field. The electret takes advantage of the ability of a fluocarbon plastic film to hold a permanent electric charge in a manner analogous to the magnetization of a permanent magnet. Although various constructions have been used, the one most widely employed uses a metal backplate having holes to reduce air stiffness. On this backplate is attached a layer of fluocarbon material (a type of teflon). Very low "bumps" are formed on the metal-fluocarbon plate, against which rests a very thin plastic diaphragm coated with a vacuum-deposited metal layer that acts as one of the microphone electrodes and that is attracted toward the charged fluocarbon film. As the diaphragm vibrates due to the action of sound waves, its distance from the charged electret varies and, following well known laws of physics, the voltage between the backplate and the diaphragm varies correspondingly. The voltage is first amplified by the field-effect transistor in the microphone and later by the hearing aid amplifier.

The electret microphone is capable of producing a very flat (i.e., high fidelity) frequency response up to frequencies well above those needed in hearing aids. Actually, it has been found to emphasize the response in the vicinity of 400 Hz in order to complement the response of receivers of the balanced armature type. The electret microphone is extremely resistant to mechanical shock and to environmental conditions, such as heat or humidity. Its most outstanding property, however, is its low sensitivity to vibration. This makes higher gain and smaller size possible in ear-level hearing aids because the microphone is 25 to 30 dB less sensitive to the mechanical vibration from the receiver, a portion of which gets back to the microphone. Thus, more gain may be used in a small hearing aid without troublesome internal mechanical feedback.

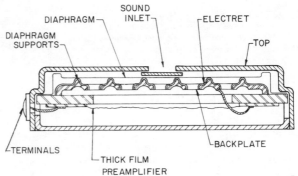

Diagram of an electret microphone used extensively in hearing aids. (Reproduced with permission of Mead C. Killion and the *Journal of the Audio Engineering Society*).

CROSS SECTION OF KNOWLES BT-1750 CONDENSER MICROPHONE

LENGTH----.312 (7.9mm)
WIDTH----.218 (5.6mm)
HEIGHT----.090(2.3mm)

Both the electret and the ceramic microphones, because of their excellent low-frequency response, have made directional microphones suitable for hearing aid use another important development of the past decade. Directional microphones have been in general use for broadcasting and public address purposes since the early 1940's and the principle of the phase-shift directional microphone has been well understood. In very small devices, the directional arrangement tends to roll off or eliminate low frequencies. It was, therefore, not too successful with magnetic microphones, which have limited low frequency response. With the ceramic or electret microphones, however, a good phase-shift design is possible. The great advantage of the directional microphone is that the ratio of speech to noise for a speaker in front of the microphone is improved because ambient noise from the rear is reduced by the directional action. Of course, the head itself has a directional effect on ear-level hearing aids, favoring sound arriving from the side of the head on which the aid is located and reducing noise effects from the opposite side. The directional microphone increases the directional effect and shifts the direction of best pickup about halfway toward the front.

Earphones

Earphones or receivers for body aids have not changed greatly in construction or performance since the significant improvements that were made in the 1940's. However, the range of sizes and responses available has increased materially. For ear-level hearing aids, the balanced armature magnetic receiver has remained the standard type, because of its high sensitivity and its susceptibility to size reduction. Available balanced-armature receivers have been markedly decreased in size in the past decade, with only minimal loss in sensitivity. Also, recently introduced types, in addition to being smaller, have wider frequency response characteristics than were formerly available.

Earmold Technology

The general concept of the custom earmold has remained valid, although materials used for earmolds have been improved and a wider selection of materials for earmolds is now available. The use of flexible silicone as an earmold material, for example, has been successful in situations where an extremely good seal to the ear canal is needed. Earmolds with a hard outer portion and a flexible canal portion (both acrylic) provide greater comfort in some cases. The basic earmold material is still hard acrylic, which combines good appearance, comfortable fit when correctly made, and easy cleanability.

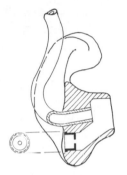

Diagram of an earmold that permits the use of different sizes of vent inserts.

The important change in earmolds in the last decade is the vastly increased use of venting, an opening in the earmold that allows passage of air into the ear canal. Today's hearing aid users are primarily persons with mild to moderate sensorineural hearing loss, for whom hearing aids work extremely well when properly fitted. Most of these persons have hearing losses that increase moderately, rapidly, or even precipitously in higher frequencies. Best results are obtained when high frequencies are amplified more than low frequencies. Adequate earmold venting is a simple and effective way to accomplish this. When venting is provided, it is also a path for the escape of sound that can get back to the microphone and cause feedback or whistling. Thus venting is not generally effective for severe hearing losses where high gain is needed.

The most radical form of venting is found in the CROS (contralateral routing of signals) and IROS (ipsilateral routing of signals) hearing aid arrangements, which have been finding wider use since their introduction, about 1965, for rapidly falling sensorineural hearing losses. In these arrangements, the earmold holds a tube that projects into the ear canal, but allows the ear canal to remain almost completely open. This permits the direct entrance of sounds that are heard well by the user, and superimposes the high-frequency sounds from the hearing aid that are needed for discrimination. The open mold causes a radical reduction in low-frequency amplification by the hearing aid, which is desirable where the hearing is nearly normal in the low-frequency range. In the CROS system, the microphone is located

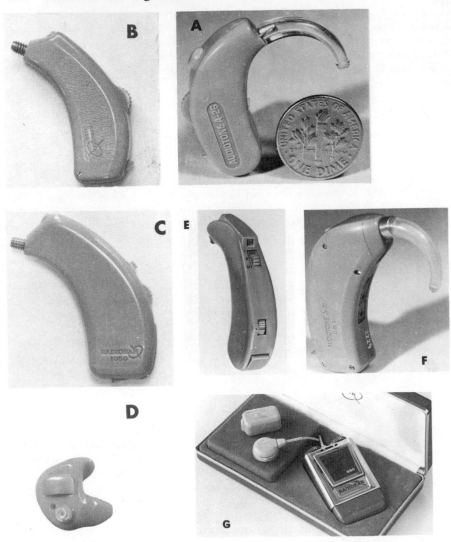

A small sampling of the many personal hearing aids currently available. Illustrations are not to a uniform scale; therefore relative size comparisons cannot be made.

A) Very tiny medium gain behind-the-ear aid, with directional microphone.

B) Small moderate gain behind-the-ear aid with several available options including AGC, extremely low current and directional microphone.

C) Small high gain, high output behind-the-ear aid with several adjustments.

D) Custom in-the-ear aid about the size of a standard earmold.

E) Small behind-the-ear aid designed for maximization of microphone directional effect.

F) Small moderate gain behind-the-ear aid with continuous adjustability of gain, frequency response, and compression.

on the opposite side of the head, to prevent feedback. In the IROS system, the gain is limited, to prevent feedback.

From the extreme of the completely open mold, varying degrees of venting are obtainable for situations requiring less low-frequency attenuation. Some types of devices allow variable venting by means of a small screw adjustment that changes the size of the opening to the outside air. Others permit adjustable venting by means of small vent inserts that can be changed by the hearing aid fitter to obtain preferred results. Then, of course, vents can be produced by drilling holes of suitable sizes in the earmold.

The important change in recent years is a better appreciation of the usefulness of venting and a better understanding of how to do it effectively.

Hearing Aid Measurement Techniques

Since the early 1940's the 2cc coupler has been used as a substitute or "standard" ear for testing hearing aid performance. While some of the shortcomings of this device have been recognized for some time, they have been more clearly defined in the last decade. For example, the 2cc coupler does not lend itself to accurate measurement of open earmold performance, such as found in CROS or in earmolds with comparatively large vents. A significant advance was made in 1970 by the development of the Zwislocki coupler, a device that resembles closely the dimensions and acoustical properties of the real ear. The effects of the head and body on hearing aid response have also been more carefully investigated. The KEMAR manikin, developed for research purposes to make more realistic measurements possible on hearing aids as they are worn, is now providing a new means of investigation. These and other developments have produced important information that will increase the meaning of hearing aid test data.

The Personal Hearing Aid in 1976

As we enter the bicentennial year of 1976, it is interesting to look again at the rate of personal hearing aid sales and the types of aids being sold. Some 463,000 aids were sold in the United States in the 12 months preceding June 30, 1975. For the first 6 months of 1975, approximately 6% were body aids, 18% were eyeglass aids, 65.6% were behind-the-ear aids, and 10.4% were in-the-ear aids. The amount of aids sold in 1975 was roughly 30% greater than in 1965, indicating a substantially increased acceptance of hearing aid help over and above that which could be attributed to the larger population.

The change in percentages of hearing aid types relative to those in 1965 is significant. Body aids have declined to about one-third of the 1965 percentage, due largely to the improved performance and greater cosmetic appeal of the ear-level aids. Even for rather severe hearing losses, powerful behind-the-ear aids are replacing body aids. Eyeglass aid percentage has dropped significantly, too, because of the greater popularity of behind-the-ear aids, which now constitute nearly two-thirds of hearing aids sold. The in-the-ear aid has advanced its position markedly within the past several years, probably because of the effectiveness of the electret microphone in reducing internal feedback and permitting greater gain in such aids. Weight and size of aids has not, on the average, changed radically in the past 10

G) High gain, high output body aid, air or bone conduction, with wide adjustability of characteristics.

Photos A and F courtesy John P. Walter and Associates and Audiotone; B, C, and G courtesy Radioear Corporation; D courtesy Starkey Laboratories, Inc.; and E courtesy Maico Hearing Instruments.

years, but more powerful aids are being put into smaller packages and tiny low-gain aids are appearing.

A Look to the Future

Looking into the future is a very uncertain business. The results of economic forecasts clearly demonstrate this. The following discussion is therefore offered only with some reservations. With respect to existing types of personal hearing aids, it is very likely that they will continue to lose market share. A hopeful direction, particularly for children's use, would be toward smaller size and extreme ruggedness. Performance characteristics should improve as better use is made of existing and future components. More compression-type body aids will probably emerge. The presently available range of adjustability should continue or increase.

Eyeglass aids will probably continue to lose some additional market share to behind-the-ear and in-the-ear aids. However, innovations in the design of eyeglass aids, such as the recently introduced wireless CROS aid, may tend to keep the eyeglass percentage higher than it would otherwise be. There is no reason to believe that the behind-the-ear aid will not remain the dominant construction for some years. The higher gains now available make it a replacement for body aids in many cases and the wide variety of characteristics available make it applicable in a large majority of cases. The greatest growth could conceivably occur in the in-the-ear category. After an earlier growth, peaking in 1966 at 9.6% of the market, the in-the-ear market share dropped to 2.3% in 1973. The share then rose to 10.4% in the first half of 1975, indicating a rather remarkable current growth rate.

With hearing aid measurements made on a more realistic basis as earlier discussed, it is probable that better hearing aid fitting techniques will develop. The recent work of Pascoe (2) and others in the United States and the earlier work of Fournier (1) in France indicate that better results are obtainable when the response curve is determined for the hearing aid as worn, and that a correction approaching a "mirror image" type of amplification may give excellent results. Continued research along this line is expected to be important.

In the near future, a new specification standard for hearing aids is likely to appear, and conformance to this will probably be asked by the Food and Drug Administration of the U.S. Department of Health, Education and Welfare. Such a standard will cause hearing aids of a given model to be more uniform in performance, since definite tolerances on a number of important characteristics will be specified. Fortunately for the hard of hearing, the proposed standard will not restrict the variety of hearing aid performance available nor inhibit advances in the state of the art.

Hearing aid costs have advanced more slowly than the cost of living and medical expenses in general. Costs usually are still considered too high by persons who have had no experience in either development, manufacture, or distribution of these tiny, labor intensive devices. It is unlikely that any major price changes will occur, particularly in consideration of increasing demands by labor and the extra costs to manufacturers and dispensers that will result from regulations expected from both the FDA and FTC. The future for the personal hearing aid does look good. If progress continues at somewhere near the rate of the past 10 years, we should certainly see happier and better communicating hearing aid users in 1986.

18   Robert Frisina, Ph.D.

Overview

The Introduction spoke to the "spirit" of the Bicentennial and its presence, felt throughout this Monograph. The chapters cover a wide range of specialities and subject matter and yet, with all the flurry of activity during the past decade, do not pretend to be exhaustive of all the possibilities. In their totality, the chapters represent an emphasis on the "social sciences" facet of deafness that was of special concern during the decade from 1965 through 1975.

As the U.S.A. celebrates its 200th anniversary, the importance of education in a free society is certain to be highlighted. A literate and informed citizenry is essential in a highly industrialized nation such as the United States. The unprecedented advances in technology during the past quarter-century present both opportunities and challenges for hearing impaired people, as they struggle to become active participants in a society where, for the most part, they have been observers.

The opportunities and challenges of today were fashioned out of a decade of rapid growth that was somewhat unharnessed and unrestrained.

- The Gross National Product of the U.S. doubled from 700 billion to nearly 1.5 trillion dollars.
- Students attending elementary and secondary schools increased in number from 40 to 45 million.
- Access to postsecondary schools rose to nearly 50% of graduating high school seniors.
- Electronics technology gave rise to computers, measurement devices, and world-wide communication networks.

The social turbulence of this first half of the past decade in general is in some ways emerging in the field of deafness. Adversary relationships fostered in the 1960's have resulted in a seeming-obsession to test the limits of our democratic system; and, for the first time in our 200-year history, two fundamental assumptions upon which this nation was founded are being challenged—first, the assumption of unlimited resources and, second, the assumption of freedom from external constraints.

It does seem that the thrust of this Monograph is positive—with skepticism voiced, yet not in strident tones. In many ways, it is a hopeful book suggesting more maturity than might characterize some of the more global features of our society.

Biomedical Highlights

The past decade has witnessed steady improvement in surgical procedures associated with middle ear anamolies. The more radical approach to remediating neurosensory deafness, although in its infancy, has begun. Research in cochlear implant electrodes with human subjects is under way. Full effect, choice of subjects, and training procedures all need to be more completely explored.

A better understanding of the genetic aspects of deafness is unfolding. Several techniques have developed that have proved to be useful in recognizing hereditary deafness syndromes; examples include the pattern of inheritance, genetic syndromes characterized by associated abnormalities, audiologic findings, and critical matings. These have been creative approaches to understanding the processes of inheritance. The longer-term and perhaps more difficult question of suggested actions regarding prevention remains to be dealt with.

Audiologic inventiveness continues to be a hallmark in the detection and diagnosis of deafness in early life. The past decade in infant hearing screening and identification audiometry might be characterized as a period of refinement. It was during this time that methodologic problems were studied, a set of guidelines were developed, and recommedations for infant hearing screening were established, including use of a high risk register with hearing screening.

Behavioral audiometry using pure tones coupled with operant conditioning principles moved forward, particularly with children who do not participate with ease in the testing situation.

Impedance audiometry in this country, in the main, was developed and tested rather broadly during the past decade. This procedure taps, in a rather direct way, the condition of the middle ear, and in so doing, adds measurably to the diagnostic inventory.

Education and Language

Teacher Preparation. The quality of instruction so vital to hearing impaired children is directly linked to the preparation of their teachers. Modern approaches to teacher preparation have their roots in the technologic advances following World War II, the members of various disciplines who became interested in the educational outcomes of deaf children, and the involvement of the federal government in educational matters. These interests of a prior decade culminated in a period of reorganization during the 1965-1975 period. A remarkable accomplishment of study, definition, adoption, and implementation of standards was completed with maximum participation of all concerned. The multifaceted ramifications of early profound deafness were recognized and attempts were made to emphasize the multidisciplinary and specialized requirements of professionals engaged in teaching deaf persons of different ages, and teaching them in a variety of educational settings.

Language and Curriculum. Linguists and psycholinguists appear very much as the "new kid on the block" in the thrust for better language development and, hence, more effective educational outcomes for deaf children and youth. Considerable work has been done during the past decade by professionals within the field of deafness and by psycholinguists outside the field. The former have concentrated on attempts to discover whether a child's language learning is developed in a delayed or in a deviant manner. Tentatively, it appears to be both, in which case deaf children develop a "dialectical" version of English similar to other dialects described by sociolinguists. Should the determination of a dialectic variation be supported through further study, a reformulation of the premises upon which current curriculum practices are based will be needed. The psycholinguists outside the field have studied "sign language" and its acquisition in deaf individuals. Their studies suggest rather strongly that the manual visuo-motor production of language may constitute a language-system base different from that produced by an auditory linguistic-based system. Another important aspect of this work in linguistics may lead sociolinguists to further clarification of the influence parent-child interaction has on acquisition of language in hearing impaired children.

Curriculum arrangements during the past decade have reflected trends in ordinary education including an emphasis on the auditory-based system of language acquisition. This results in part from improved measurement of hearing that indicates that 90% of all children with educationally significant hearing impairment are likely to receive some benefit if amplification is used early and consistently. Also, the auditory-based approach in part is due to advances that have been made in the performance and availability of wearable hearing aids as well as other special types of equipment and teaching methodologies. Individualized instruction, open classrooms, integrated classrooms, instructional technology,and modernized versions of what historically has been known as the natural method of language learning are being utilized and evaluated.

Instructional Settings and Practices. The decade of the 1960's reopened the debate regarding the melting pot theory of America, first advanced as different ethnic immigrants reached its shores. In the case of Blacks and some other groups, it is probably more accurate to describe America as a salad bowl rather than a melting pot; each group unique unto itself and at the same time reaching out to common beliefs, hopes, and aspirations.

Other socio-political concepts introduced have included egalitarian, equalitarian, individual rights, and most recently in the case of handicapped children, least restrictive environment. In association with heavy urbanization, modern transportation and legal thrusts during the past decade, education in one's community is becoming more commonplace. Mainstreaming or integrated education are terms associated with programs for hearing impaired children. As a result, instructional settings of a wide variety now exist for infants and children of 2 and 3 years of age all the way to organized postsecondary efforts. Although integrated programs have been operating in a few places for at least a decade, the variety and quantity of such efforts are more widespread at present than any time in the past. Availability of professional personnel, funding, acceptance by regular educators, and appropriate research will be needed to implement an intelligent program appropriate to each child's needs and educational rights.

Irrespective of the setting, several instructional practices have been on scene during the 1965-1975 period. The two that have been given the greatest visibility are the auditory-oral and the total communication approaches. Both use the auditory-based linguistic model. As practiced by some, the former frequently underemphasizes the role of vision, while the latter often underemphasizes the role of audition. The methods referred to as "visual-oral" and "visible English" round out the spectrum of instructional communication practices in use today. Comprehensive research is sorely needed to determine which methods should be used with which children and when.

Communication Technology. The profession entered the 1965-1975 decade with considerable experience in the use of amplification. Wearable hearing aids and auditory training that were readily available in large part were aided by a new thrust in federal funding. The steady improvement in design and quality of wearable hearing aids with a continuing diminution in size has made it possible for even those with severe and profound deafness to change from body-worn to ear-level instruments. New microphones and receivers and improved power requirements, along with other technical advances, have made the dramatic shift in size feasible without seriously affecting frequency response and gain characteristics. However, sole reliance on audition for language acquisition in early profound deafness, or any other unilateral approach, is not suggested by the data in hand.

Concurrent with miniaturization of hearing aids and the federal investment in education during the past decade have been advances in availability of sensory aids in addition to hearing aids. Visual speech feedback devices, although still in the experimental stage, are relatively well-developed and available for those programs that have the interest and the personnel to use them. Vibratory and tactile devices, on the other hand, are not well developed nor tested to any extent approaching their potential effectiveness with persons who are profoundly deaf.

Instructional and learning aids, largely due to the pioneering of the Captioned Films Program for the Deaf, resulted in overhead transparencies, films and television becoming commonplace in schools and classes for hearing impaired children throughout the U.S.A. In spite of all these efforts, the field still falls short of much-needed empirical data regarding graphic communication. How best to caption and graphically display printed material via TV and film remains virtually unexplored. Only a few studies have been completed while others are currently underway.

Alexander Graham Bell invented the telephone 100 years ago. It was not until the decade under study that it was capitalized on for use by deaf people. Coupled to a pair of teletypewriters (TTY) the telephone becomes the transmission link between them. Networks among hearing impaired persons and others are now being developed in a number of cities. Uses for social, business, and emergency purposes are now available although perhaps not on as large a scale as might be desirable. This advance, nonetheless, represents a most significant breakthrough during the past decade.

Psycho-Social and Rehabilitation Services. In this monograph, strengths and weaknesses in the delivery of services for hearing impaired persons are articulated in a number of ways. The reader is reminded on more than one occasion that the self-study of any service provider can be a healthy activity. A prominent departure in the psycho-social areas is the advocacy role being assumed. Contributions to research, community service, and training have taken on new enthusiasm. The work of many is recognized and the reader is cautioned against concluding for all time on the basis of what data are presently in. A warning is given against overgeneralizing from statistical differences that may be of limited or no practical significance. Interestingly, the work of some psychologists is extending the "just find out" stage into the program implementation phase. Care must be taken, however, when an advocacy posture is taken. The question in such a circumstance is whether or not the advocacy role affects one's objectivity, and hence results in a continuation of designated shortcomings of others, only in a new form.

For the first time, comprehensive demographic data through a national population study became available during the latter part of the past decade. Also, noteworthy accomplishments occurred in mobilizing community resources, and, in several states, commissions on deafness were established. However, cross-talk between and among disciplines in the social, behavorial, and health sciences needs to be improved if more is to be achieved with the same or fewer resources in the decade that follows. There is faint hope that the proliferation of legislation in education and social services of the last decade will likely be repeated during the next. Gains to be made will require an unprecedented persuasion, productivity, and accountability that will test even the heartiest among us. Some advances might come in the broadening of health and education legislation that presently does not include "the handicapped."

International exchanges through generous government support seem to be a thing of the past. Imaginative purposes will be required in order to reestablish the steady flow of people across national boundaries that so characterized the last decade.

All in all, the 1965-1975 period contained within it the peak of widespread government spending in research, demonstration, and training, in education, health, and welfare. Much learning and sharing took place, but often in somewhat undisciplined ways. The social upheaval reflected in the cities and on the campuses attained its high watermark during this period. Retrenchment is the order of the day in many quarters. Yet, in the case of deaf children whose ages at onset are steadily moving closer to birth, there cannot be a relaxation of effort, enthusiasm, or inventiveness.

For deaf persons and those who toil on their behalf, paraphrasing Thomas Wolfe should remind us all of the unfinished business and its importance ... If a deaf person has a talent and cannot use it, we have failed. If a deaf person has a talent and uses only half of it, we have partly failed. If a deaf person has a talent and learns somehow to use the whole of it, he (and we) have gloriously succeeded, and won satisfaction and a triumph few people ever know.   ⚠

Chapter 1

1. Goode, R. L. Personal communication, Stanford University.
2. Fisch, U. Personal communication, Zurich, Switzerland.
3. House, W. F. Symposium on cochlear implants, I.: Goals of the cochlear implant. *Laryngoscope*, 1974, *84*, 1883-1887.
4. Linthicum, F.H. Evauation of the child with a sensorineural hearing impairment. *Otolaryngol Clin N. Am.*, 1975, *8*, 69-75.
5. Shambaugh, G.E., Causse, J., Petrovic, A. Chevance, L. G., & Valvassouri, G.E. New concepts in the management of otospongiosis. *Arch Otolaryngol*, 1975, *100*, 419-426.

Chapter 2

1. Conneally, P.M., Rose, S.P., Fox, P.B., & Nance, W.E. Genetic analysis of pedigree data from a nationwide survey of deaf children. *Am. J. Hum. Genet.*, 1975, *27*, 27a.
2. Fay, E.A. *Marriages of deaf in America*. Washington, D.C.: The Volta Bureau. 1898, pp. 1-527.
3. Fraser, G.R. Association of congenital deafness with goitre. *Ann. Hum. Genet.* 1965, *28*, 201-249.
4. Fraser, G.R., Froggatt, P., & James, T.N. Congenital deafness associated with electrocardiographic abnormalities, fainting attacks and sudden death. *Quart. J. Med.*, 1964, *33*, 361-385.
5. Fraser, G.R., Froggatt, P., & Murphy, T. Genetic aspects of the cardio-auditory syndrome of Hervell and Lange-Nielsen (congenital deafness and electrocardiographic abnormalities). *Ann. Hum. Genet.*, 1964, *28*, 133-157.
6. Nance, W.E., & McConnell, F.E. Status and prospects of research in hereditary deafness. *Adv. Hum. Genet.*, 1973, *4*, 173-250.
7. Nance, W.E., Rose, S., Conneally, P.M., & Miller, J. Opportunities for genetic counseling through institutional ascertainment of affected probands. *Proceedings of a Conference on Genetic Counseling*, in press.
8. Nance, W.E., Rose, S., Prokach, A., & Conneally, P.M. The use of pedigree linkage for the diagnosis of hereditary deafness. *Am. J. Hum. Genet.*, 1975, *27*, 68a.
9. Nance, W.E., & Sweeney, A. Genetic factors in deafness of early life. *Otol. Clin. N. Amer.*, 1975, *8*, 19-48.
10. Preus, M., & Fraser, F.C. Genetics of hereditary nephropathy with deafness (Alport's syndrome). *Clin. Genet.*, 1971, *2*, 331-337.
11. Rose, S.P. *Genetic studies of profound prelingual deafness*. Unpublished doctoral dissertation, Indiana University, 1975.
12. Rose, S.P., Nance, W.E., Hughes, E., & Conneally, P.M. Genetic analysis of profound prelingual deafness. *Am. J. Hum. Genet.*, 1975, *27*, 78a.
13. Steinberg, D. The metabolic basis of Refsum syndrome. *Birth Defects Orig. Art. Ser.*, 1971, *7*, 42-52.
14. Stewart, J., & Bergstrom, L. Familial hand abnormality and sensorineural deafness: A new syndrome. *J. Pediat.*, 1971, *78*, 102-110.
15. Vanderbilt University Hereditary Deafness Study Group. Dominantly inherited low-frequency hearing loss. *Arch. Otolaryngol.*, 1968, *88*, 242-250.
16. Vernon, M. Usher's syndrome—Deafness and progressive blindness: Clinical cases, prevention and literature survey.*J. Chron. Dis.*, 1969, *22*, 133.
17. Vernon, M. Overview of Usher's syndrome: Congenital deafness and progressive loss of vision. *Volta Rev.*, 1974, *76*, 100.
18. Waardenburg, P.J. A new syndrome combining developmental anomalies of the eyelids, eyebrows and nose root with pigmentary defects of the iris and head hair and with congenital deafness. *Am. J. Hum. Genet.*, 1951, *3*, 195-253.
19. Ziprkowksi, L., Krakowski, A., Adam, A., Costeff, H., & Sade, J. Partial albinism and deafmutism. *Arch. Dermat.*, 1962, *86*, 530-539.

Chapter 3

1. AAOO, AAP, ASHA. Committee statement on infant hearing screening. *Asha*, 1971, *13*, 79.

2. AAOO, AAP, & ASHA. Supplementary statement of the joint committee on infant hearing screening. *Asha*, 1974, *16*, 160.
3. Alberti, P.W., & Kristensen, R. The clinical application of impedance audiometry. *Laryngoscope*, 1970, *80*, 735-746.
4. Guidelines for identification audiometry. *Asha*, 1975, *17*, 94-99.
5. Barr, B. Pure tone audiometry for preschool children. *Acta Oto-Laryngol., Suppl.*, 1955, *121*, 1-84.
6. Bartoshuk, A.D. Human neonatal cardiac acceleration to sound: Habituation and dishabituation. *Percept. Motor Skills*, 1962, *15*, 15-27.
7. Bartoshuk, A.K. Human neonatal cardiac responses to sound: A power function. *Psychonomic Sci.*, 1964, *1*, 151-152.
8. Bench, J., Hoffman, E., & Wilson, I. A comparison of live and videorecord viewing of infant behavior under sound stimulation. *Develpm. Psychobiol.*, 1974, *7*, 455-464.
9. Berlin, C.I., & Cullen, J.K. The physical basis of impedance measurement. In J. Jerger. (Ed.), *Handbook of clinical impedance audiometry*. Dobbs Ferry, N.Y.: Morgan Press, 1974, pp. 1-20.
10. Berlin, C.I., Cullen, J.K., Ellis, M.S., Lousteau, R.J., Yarbrough, W.M., & Lyons, G.D. Clinical application of recording human VIIIth nerve action potentials from the tympanic membrane *Transactions Am. Acad. Ophthalmol. Otolaryngol*, 1974, *78*, 401-410.
11. Berlin, C., & Lowe, S. Temporal and dichotic factors in central auditory & testing. In J. Katz. (Ed.), *Handbook of clinical audiology*. Baltimore: Williams & Wilkins, 1972, pp. 280-312.
12. Blank, M Cognitive processes in auditory discrimination in normal and retarded readers. *Child Develpm.*, 1968, *39*, 1091-1101.
13. Bluestone, C.D., Beery, Q.C., & Paradise, J.L. Audiometry and tympanometry in relation to middle ear effusions in children. *Laryngoscope*, 1973, *83*, 594-603.
14. Bradford, L., & Rousey, C. *Respiration audiometry* (Report 6). Minneapolis: Maico Audiological Library Series, 10, 1972.
15. Bradford, L.J. Respiration audiometry; the indirect assessment of hearing sensitivity. *Audiol. Hearing Educ.*, 1975, *1*, 19-25.
16. Bricker, D.D., & Bricker, W.A. A programmed approach to operant audiology for low-functioning children. *J. Speech Hearing Dis.*, 1969(a), *34*, 312-320.
17. Bricker, W.A., & Bricker, D.D. Four operant procedures for establishing auditory stimulus control with low-functioning children. *Am. J. Mental Deficiency*, 1969(b), *73*, 981-987.
18. Brooks, D.N. An objective method of detecting fluid in the middle ear. *Internat. Audiol.*, 1968, *7*, 280.
19. Brooks, D.N. The use of the electro-acoustic impedance bridge in the assessment of middle ear function. *Internat. Audiol.*, 1969, *8*, 563-569.
20. Brooks, D.N. Electro-acoustic impedance bridge studies on normal ears of children. *J. Speech Hearing Res.*, 1971, *14*, 247-253.
21. Brooks, D.N. Impedance measurement in screening for auditory disorders in children. *Hearing Instruments*, 1974, *36*, 20-21.
22. Buktenica, N.A. *Test of nonverbal auditory discrimination* (TENVAD). Chicago: Follett Publishing Co., 1975.
23. Butler, K. *Auditory Figure Ground Test (AFGT)*. Cupertino, Ca., 1974. (Avail. from author)
24. Butterfield, G.A. Note on the use of cardiac rate in the audiometric appraisal of retarded children. *J. Speech Hearing Dis.* 1962, *27*, 378-379.
25. Butterfield, E.C., & Cairns, S.F. Summary-infant reception research. In R.L. Schiefelbusch, & L.L. Lloyd (Eds.), *Language perspectives-Acquisition, retardation, and intervention*. Baltimore: University Park Press, 1974, pp. 75-84.
26. Butterfield, E.C., & Siperstein, G.N. Influence of contingent auditory stimulation upon non-nutritional suckle. In J. Bosma (Ed.), *Oral sensation and perception: The mouth of the infant*. Springfield, Il: Charles C Thomas, 1973.
27. Campanelli, P. A measure of intra-list stability of four PAL word lists. *J. Audi. Res.*, 1962, *2*, 50-55.
28. Campbell, R. Discrimination test word difficulty. *J. Speech Hearing Res.*, 1965, *8*, 13-22.
29. Clifton, R.K., & Meyers, W.J. The heart-rate response of four-month-old infants to auditory stimuli. *J. Exper. Child Psychol.*, 1969, *7*, 122-135.
30. Cohn, R. Differential cerebral dominance to noise and verbal stimuli. *Transactions Am. Neurolog. Assoc.*, 1971, *96*, 127-131.

31. Collyer, Y., Bench, J., & Wilson, I. Newborns' responses to auditory stimuli judged in relation to stimulus onset and offset. *Brit. J. Audiol.*, 1974, *8*, 14-17.
32. Crum, P. A comparison of the validity and reliability of the puretone and verbal auditory screening (VASC) tests for normal hearing and selected hearing impaired groups (Unpublished master's thesis). University of Alabama, 1972.
33. Cullen, J.K., Ellis, M.S., Berlin, C.I., & Lousteau, R.J. Human acoustic nerve action potential recordings from the tympanic membrane without anesthesia. *Acta Oto-Laryngol.*, 1972, *74*, 15-22.
34. Cunningham, G.C. *Conference on newborn hearing screening.* California State Department of Public Health, Berkeley; and Public Health Service, HEW, Rockville, Md., 1971.
35. Dahle, A.J. *Comparison of the verbal auditory screening for children (VASC) tests and pure tone tests in screening the hearing of mentally retarded children.* Southeast American Association on Mental Deficiency Annual Convention, Nashville, Tn. 1972.
36. Dahle, A.J., & Daly, D.A. Tangible rewards in assessing auditory discrimination performance of mentally retarded children. *Am. J. Mental Deficiency*, 1974, *78*, 625-630.
37. Dahle, A.J., McCollister, F.P., Hammer, B.A., Reynolds, D.W., & Stagno, W. Subclinical congenital cytomegalovirus infection and hearing impairment. *J. Speech Hearing Dis.*, 1974, *39*, 320-329.
38. Daly, R.L. Peripheral vasoconstriction and electroencephalography as estimators of hearing threshold. *Asha*, 1965, *7*, 419. (Abstract)
39. Dansinger, S., & Madow, A.A. Verbal auditory screening with the mentally retarded. *Am. J. Mental Deficiency*, 1966, *71*, 387-392.
40. Darley, F.L. Identification audiometry. *J. Speech Hearing Dis.*, Monog. Suppl. #9, 1961.
41. Davis, P.A. Effects of acoustic stimuli on the waking human brain. *J. Neurophysiol.*, 1939, *2*, 494-499.
42. Davis, H. The young deaf child: Identification and management. *Acta Oto-Laryngol.*, 1965, Suppl. 206, pp. 33-52.
43. Davis, H. Averaged evoked response EEG audiometry in North America. *Acta Oto-Laryngol.*, 1968, *65*, 79-85.
44. Derbyshire, A.J., & Davis, H. The action potential of the auditory nerve *Am. J. Physiol.*, 1935, *113*, 476-504.
45. DiCarlo, L., & Bradley, W. A simplified test for infants and young children. *Laryngoscope*, 1961, *71*, 628-646.
46. Dix, M.R., & Hallpike, C.S. The peepshow: A new technique for pure-tone audiometry in young children. *Brit. Med. J.*, 1947, *2*, 719-723.
47. Downs, M.P. Audiometry in children. *Internat. Audiol.*, 1947, *1*, 268-270.
48. Downs, M.P., & Hemenway, W.G. Newborn screening revisited. *Hearing Speech News*, 1972, *40*, 4-5; 26; 28-29.
49. Downs, M.P., & Silver, H.K. The A.B.D.C.'s to H.E.A.R. *Clin. Pediat.*, 1972, *10*, 563-566.
50. Downs, M.P., & Sterritt, G.M. Identification audiometry for neonates: A preliminary report. *J. Aud. Res.*, 1964, *4*, 69-80.
51. Egan, J.P. *Articulation testing methods* (OSRD Report 3802). Washington, D.C.: U.S. Dept. Comm., Off. Tech. Serv., 1944.
52. Eilers, R.E., Wilson, W.R., & Moore, J.M. Developmental changes in infant speech perception. In preparation.
53. Eimas, P.D. Linguistic processing of speech by young infants. In R.L. Schiefelbusch & L.L. Lloyd (Eds.), *Language perspectives - acquisition, retardation and intervention.* Baltimore: University Park Press, 1974, pp. 55-73.
54. Eimas, P.D., Siqueland, E.R., Juoczyk, P., & Vigorito, J. Speech perception in infants. *Science*, 1971, *171*, 303-306.
55. Eisele, W.A., Berry, R.C., & Shriner, T.H. Infant sucking response patterns as a conjugate function of changes in the sound pressure level of auditory stimuli. *J. Speech Hearing Res.*, 1975, *18*, 296-307.
56. Eisenberg, R.B., Auditory behavior in the human neonate: I. Methodologic problems and the logical design of research procedures. *J. Aud. Res.*, 1965, *5*, 159-177.
57. Eisenberg, R.B. Auditory competence in early life: The roots of communicative behavior. Baltimore: University Park Press, 1976.
58. Evans, M.L. An adaptation of audiometric technique for use with small children. Unpublished master's thesis, University of Illinois, 1943.
59. Fairbanks, R. The rhyme test: A test of discrimination. *J. Acoust. Soc. Am.*, 1958, *30*, 596-600.

60. Fletcher, H. The nature of speech and its interpretation. *Bell Sys. Tech. Jour.*, 1922, 129-144.
61. Flowers, A. *Flowers auditory test of selective attention (FATSA)*. Dearborn, Mi: Percept. Learning Sy., 1975(a).
62. Flowers, A. *Short term auditory retrieval and storage test (STARS)*. Dearborn, Mi: Percept. Learning Sys. 1975(b).
63. Frisina, R. Audiometric evaluation and its relation to habilitation and rehabilitation of the deaf. *Am. Ann. Deaf*, 1962, *107*, 478-481.
64. Frisina, R. Measurement of hearing in children. In J. Jerger (Ed.), *Modern development in audiology*. New York: Academic Press, 1963, pp. 126-166.
65. Fristoe, M. *Language intervention systems for the retarded: A catalog of original structured language programs in use in the U.S*. Montgomery: State of Alabama Dept. of Educ., 1975.
66. Fudula, J., Kunze, L.H., & Ross, J.D. *Auditory Pointing Test*. San Rafael, Ca.: Academic Therapy Publ., 1974.
67. Fulton, R.T. *Auditory stimulus-response control*. Baltimore: University Park Press, 1964.
68. Fulton, R., & Lamb, L. Acoustic impedance and tympanometry with the retarded: A normative study. *Audiology*, 1972, *11*, 199-208.
69. Fulton, R.T., & Lloyd, L.L. *Auditory assessment of the difficult-to-test*. Baltimore: Williams & Wilkins, 1975.
70. Galambos, C.S., & Galambos, R. Brain stem auditory-evoked responses in premature infants. *J. Speech Hearing Res.*, 1975, *18*, 456-465.
71. Gerwin, K.S., & Glorig, A. *Detection of hearing loss and ear disease in children*. Springfield, Il.: Charles C Thomas, 1974.
72. Glorig, A. Routine neonate hearing. *Hearing Speech News*, 1971, *4*, 7.
73. Goldman, R., Fristoe, M., & Woodcock, R. *G-F-W test of auditory discrimination*. Circle Pines, Mn.: Am. Guid. Serv., 1970.
74. Goldman, R., Fristoe, M. & Woodcock, R. *G-F-W auditory skills test battery*. Circle Pines, Mn.: Am. Guid. Serv., 1974(a).
75. Goldman, R., Fristoe, M., & Woodcock, R. *G-F-W diagnostic auditory discrimination test*. Circle Pines, Mn.: Am. Guid. Serv., 1974(b).
76. Goldstein, R. Electrophysiologic audiometry. In J. Jerger (Ed.), *Modern developments in audiology*. New York: Academic Press, 1963, pp. 167-192.
77. Goldstein, R. Electroencephalic audiometry. In J. Jerger (Ed.), *Modern developments in audiology* (2nd ed.). New York: Academic Press, 1973, pp. 407-433.
78. Goldstein, R., & Rodman, L.B. Early components of averaged evoked responses to rapidly repeated auditory stimuli. *J. Speech Hearing Res.*, 1967, *10*, 697-705.
79. Goldstein, R., & Tait, C. Critique of neonatal hearing evaluation. *J. Speech Hearing Dis.*, 1971, *36*, 3-18.
80. Goodman, W.S., Appleby, S.V., Scott, J.W., & Ireland, P.E. Audiometry in newborn children by electroencephalography. *Laryngoscope*, 1964, *74*, 1316-1328.
81. Griffing, T., Simonton, K., & Hedgecock, L.D. Verbal auditory screening for children. *Minnesota Med.*, 1962, *45*, 34-36.
82. Griffing, T., Simonton, K.M., & Hedgecock, L.D. Verbal auditory screening for preschool children. *Transaction Am. Acad. Ophthalmol. Otolaryngol.*, 1967, *71*, 105-111.
83. Hardy, J.B. Fetal consequences of maternal viral infections in pregnancy. *Arch. Otolaryngol.*, 1973, *98*, 218-227.
84. Hardy, J.B., Dougherty, A., & Hardy, W.G. Hearing responses and audiologic screening in infants. *J. Pediat.*, 1959, *55*, 382-390.
85. Hardy, W.G., & Pauls, M.D. The test situation of PGSR audiometry. *J. Speech Hearing Dis.*, 1952, *17*, 13-24.
86. Hartman, E.E. Screening preschool children for hearing loss. *Minnesota Med.* 1965, *48*, 527-529.
87. Haskins, H. *A phonetically balanced test of speech discrimination for children*. Master's thesis, Northwestern University, 1949.
88. Hirsh, I., Davis, H., Silverman, S., Reynolds, E., Eldert, E., & Benson, R. Development of materials for speech and audiometry. *J. Speech Hearing Dis.*, 1952, *17*, 321-337.
89. Hodgson, W.R. Filtered speech tests. In J. Katz (Ed.), *Handbook of clinical audiology*. Baltimore: Williams & Wilkins, 1972, pp. 313-324.
90. Hogan, D.D. Autonomic correlates of audition. In R.E. Fulton, & L.L. Lloyd (Eds.), *Auditory assessment of the difficult-to-test*. Baltimore: Williams & Wilkins, 1965, pp. 262-290.

91. House, A.S., Williams, C.E., Hecker, M.H.L., & Kryter, K.D. Articulation testing methods: Consonantal differentiation with a closed-response set. *J. Acoust. Soc. Am.*, 1965, *37*, 158-166.
92. Hudgins, C., & Numbers, M. Speech perception in present day education for deaf children. *Volta Rev.*, 1948, *50*, 449-456.
93. Huizing, H. *Proceedings of the International Course of Paedo-Audiology*, Groningen, *88*, 1953.
94. Irwin, J.V., Hind, J.E., & Aronson, A.E. Experience with condition GSR audiometry in a group of mentally deficient individuals. *Training Sch. Bull.* 1957, *54*, 26-31.
95. Jerger, J. Clinical experience with impedance audiometry. *Arch. Oto-Laryngol.*, 1970, *92*, 311-324.
96. Jerger, J. *Handbook of clinical impedance audiometry*. Dobbs Ferry, N.Y.: Morgan Press, 1975, pp. 149-174.
97. Jerger, J., Burney, P., Mauldin, L., & Crump, B. Predicting hearing loss from the acoustic reflex. *J. Speech Hearing Dis.*, 1974, *39*, 1.
98. Jewett, D.L., & Williston, J.S. Auditory-evoked far fields averaged from the scalp of humans. *Brain*, 1971, *94*, 681-696.
99. Katz, J. *Kindergarten auditory screening test, parts I and II*. Chicago: Follett Educ. Corp., 1971.
100. Katz, J. *Staggered spondaic word (SSW) test*. Brentwood, Mo.: Auditec, 1973.
101. Keith, R.W. Impedance audiometry with neonates. *Arch. Otolaryngol.*, 1973, *97*, 465-467.
102. Kelemen, G. Toxoplasmosis and congenital deafness. A.M.A. *Arch. Otolaryngol.* 1958, *68*, 547-561.
103. Knox, A.W. Electrodermal audiometry. In J. Katz (Ed.), *Handbook of clinical audiology*, Baltimore: Williams & Wilkins, 1972, pp. 395-406.
104. Knox, E.C. A method of obtaining pure tone audiograms in young children. *J. Laryngol. Otol.*, 1960, *74*, 475-479.
105. Kodman, F., Fein, A., & Mixon, A. Psychogalvanic skin response audiometry with severe mentally retarded children. *Am. J. Mental Deficiency*, 1959, *64*, 131-136.
106. Kryter, K.D., & Whitman, E.C. Some comparison between rhyme and PB-word intelligibility tests. *J. Acoust. Soc. Am.*, 1965, *37*, 1146.
107. Lamb, L.E., & Norris, T.W. Acoustic impedance measurement. In R.T. Fulton, & L.L. Lloyd (Eds.), *Audiometry for the retarded*. Baltimore: Williams & Wilkins, 1969, pp. 164-209.
108. Lamb, L.E., & Norris, T.W. Relative acoustic impedance measurements with mentally retarded children. *Am. J. Mental Deficiency*, 1970, *75*, 51-56.
109. Langford, C., Bench, J., & Wilson, I. Some effects of prestimulus activity and length of prestimulus observation on judgments of newborns' responses to sounds. *Audiology*, 1975, *14*, 44-52.
110. Lindsay, J.R. Histopathology of deafness due to postnatal viral disease. *Arch. Otolaryngol.*, 1973, *98*, 258-264.
111. Ling, D., Ling, A.H., & Doehring, D.C. Stimulus, response and observer variables in the auditory screening of newborn infants. *J. Speech Hearing Res.*, 1970, *13*, 9-18.
112. Lloyd, L.L. The use of the slide show audiometric technique with mentally retarded children. *Except. Child.*, 1965(d), *32*, 93-98.
113. Lloyd, L.L. Comparisons of six selected audiometric measures on retarded children: A preliminary report. In L.L. Lloyd & D.R. Frisina (Eds.), *The audiologic assessment of the mentally retarded: Proceedings of a national conference*. Parsons, Ks.: Speech and Hearing Dept., Parsons State Hospital Training Cr., 1965(b), pp. 99-118.
114. Lloyd, L.L. Behavioral audiometry viewed as an operant procedure. *J. Speech Hearing Dis.*, 1966, *31*, 128-136.
115. Lloyd, L.L. Behavioral audiometry with children. In E.L. Eagles (Ed.), *Human communications and its disorders* (Vol. 3 of *The nervous system*). New York: Raven Press, 1975(a), pp. 173-179.
116. Lloyd, L.L. Discussants comment: Language and communication aspects. In T.D. Tjossem (Ed.), *Intervention strategies for high risk infants and young children*. Baltimore: University Park Press, in press.
117. Lloyd, L.L., & Cox, B.P. Behavioral audiometry with children. In M.J. Glasscock (Guest Ed.), *The otolaryngology clinics of North America: Symposium on sensorineural hearing loss in children: Early detection and intervention*. Philadelphia: W.B. Saunders, 1975(b), pp. 89-107.

118. Lloyd, L.L., & Frisina, R. *The audiologic assessment of the mentally retarded proceedings of a national conference.* Parsons, Ks.: Speech Hearing Dept., Parsons State Hosp. Training Cr., 1965.

119. Lloyd, L.L., & Melrose, J. Inter-method comparisons of selected audiometric measures used with normal hearing mentally retarded children. *J. Aud. Res.*, 1966, 6, 205-217.

120. Lloyd, L.L., & Wilson, W.R. Recent developments in the behavioral assessment of the infant's response to auditory stimulation. *Proceedings of the XVI World Congress for Logopedics and Phoniatrics,* Interlaken, Switzerland, 1974.

121. Lloyd, L.L., Spradlin, J.E., & Reid, M.J. An operant audiometric procedure for difficult-to-test patients. *J. Speech Hearing Dis.*, 1968, 33, 236-245.

122. Lowell, E., Rushford, G., Hoversten, G., & Stoner, M. Evaluation of pure tone audiometry with preschool age children. *J. Speech Hearing Dis.*, 1956, 21, 292-302.

123. Lowell, M.O., Lowell, E.L., & Goodhill, V. Evoked response audiometry with infants: A longitudinal study. *Audiol. Hearing Educ.*, 1975, 1, 32-37.

124. McAdam, D.W., & Whitaker, H.A. Language production: Electroencephalographic localization in the normal human brain. *Science*, 1971, 172, 499.

125. McCandless, G.A. Clinical application of evoked response audiometry. *J. Speech Hearing Res.*, 1967, 10 468-478.

126. McCandless, G.A. Future directions. In J. Jerger (Ed.), *Handbook of clinical impedance audiometry.* Dobbs Ferry, N.Y.: Morgan Press, 1975, pp. 175-188.

127. McCandless, G.A. & Thomas, G.K. Impedance audiometry as a screening procedure for middle ear disease. *Transactions Am. Acad. Ophthalmol. Otolaryngol.*, 1974, 78, 98-102.

128. Mecham, M., Jex, J., & Jones, J. *Tests of listening accuracy in children.* Salt Lake City, Ut.: Communic. Res. Assoc., 1974.

129. Mencher, G.T. Screening infants for auditory deficits: University of Nebraska neonatal hearing project. *J. Aud. Communic.*, (Supplement 11), 1972.

130. Mencher, G.T. *Infant hearing screening: The state of the art.* Minneapolis: Maico Audiological Library Series, 1974, 12, #7.

131. Metz, O. The acoustic impedance measured on normal and pathological ears. *Acta Otolaryngol.*, (Suppl. 63), 1946.

132. Meyerson, L., & Michael, J.L. *The measurement of sensory thresholds in exceptional children: An experimental approach to some problems of differential diagnosis and education with special reference to hearing* (OE-HEW Coop. Res. Proj. #418), Houston, Tx.: University of Houston, 1960.

133. Meyerson, L., & Michael, J.L. Assessment of hearing by operant conditioning procedures. In *Report of the proceedings of the international congress on education of the deaf and of the 41st meeting of the convention of American Instructors of the Deaf.* Washington, D.C.: U.S. Govt. Printing Off., 1964, pp. 236-242.

134. Mills, P.J., Derbyshire, A.J., & Carter, R.L. Changes evoked by auditory stimulation in the EEG in sleep. *Electroencephalog. Clin. Neurophysiol.*, 1961, 13, 79-90.

135. Moffit, A.R. Consonant cue perception by twenty to twenty-four-week-old infants. *Child Developm.*, 1971, 42, 717-731.

136. Molofese, D.L. *Cerebral asymmetry in infants, children and adults: Auditory evoked responses to speech and noise stimuli.* Doctoral dissertation. Penn State University. 1972, University Document #73-20; 105, University Microfilms, Ann Arbor, Mi.

137. Moncur, J.P. Judge reliability in infant testing. *J. Speech Hearing Res.*, 1968, 11, 348-357.

138. Moore, J.M., Thompson, G., & Thompson, M. Auditory localization of infants as a function of reinforcement conditions. *J. Speech Hearing Dis.* 1975, 40, 29-34.

139. Moore, J.M., Wilson, W.R., & Thompson, G. Visual reinforcement of head-turn responses in infants under twelve months of age. In preparation.

140. Morrell, L.K., & Huntington, D.A. Electrocortical localization of language production. *Science*, 1971, 174, 1359-1360.

141. Morse, P.A. Infant speech perception: A preliminary model and review of the literature. In R.L. Schiefelbusch & L.L. Lloyd (Eds.), *Language perspectives - Acquisition, retardation and intervention.* Baltimore: University Park Press, 1974, pp. 19-48.

142. Murphy, K.P. Development of hearing in babies. *Child and Family*, 1962, 1, 16-17.

143. Myatt, B., & Landers, B. Assessing discrimination loss in children. *Arch. Otolaryngol.*, 1963, 77, 359-362.

144. Nasca, F. An investigation of the PICSI test: Picture identification for children; a standard index. *Dissert. Abst.*, 1964, 28, 1218.

145. Newby, H.A. *Audiology.* New York: Appleton-Century-Crofts, 1964.
146. Nickerson, J.F., Miller, A.W., & Shyne, N.A. *A comparison of five articulation tests.* Bozeman, Mt.: Electron. Res. Lab., Montana St. Coll., 1960.
147. Niemeyer, W., & Sesterhenn. Calculating the hearing threshold from the stapedius reflex threshold for different sound stimuli. *Audiology,* 1974, *13,* 421-427.
148. Northern, J.L., & Downs, M.P. *Hearing in children.* Baltimore: Williams & Wilkins, 1974.
149. O'Neill, J., Oyer, H.J., & Hillis, J.W. Audiometric procedures used with children. *J. Speech Hearing Dis.,* 1961, *26,* 61-66.
150. Peckham, C.S. Clinical and laboratory study of children exposed in utero to maternal rubella. *Arch. Disease Childhood,* 1972, *47,* 571-577.
151. Peronnet, F., Michel, F., Echallier, J.F., & Girod, J. Coronal topography of human audiotry evoked response. *Electroencephalog. Clin. Neurophysiol.,* 1974, *37,* 225-230.
152. Picton, T.W., Hillyard, S.A., Krausz, H.I., & Galambos, R. Human auditory evoked potentials, I: Evaluation of components. *Electroencephalog. Clin. Neurophysiol.,* 1974, *30,* 179-190.
153. Price, L.L. Evoked response audiometry. In R.T. Fulton & L.L. Lloyd, (Eds.), *Auditory assessment of the difficult-to-test.* Baltimore: Williams & Wilkins, 1975, pp. 235-261.
154. Pronovost, W., & Dumbleton, C. Boston University speech sound discrimination picture test. Boston: Boston University, 1953.
155. Reneau, J.P., & Hnatiow, G.Z. Evoked response audiometry: A topical and historical review. Baltimore: University Park Press, 1975.
156. Reynolds, D.W., Stagno, S., Stubbs, K.G., Dahle, A.J., Saxon, S.A., & Alford, C.A. Inapparent congenital cytomegalovirus infection: Casual relationship with auditory and mental deficiency. *New Eng. J. Med.,* 1974, *290,* 291-296.
157. Ritchie, B.C., & Merklein, R.A. An evaluation of the efficiency of the verbal auditory screening for children (VASC). *J. Speech Hearing Res.,* 1972, *15,* 280-286.
158. Robertson, E.O., Peterson, J.L., & Lamb, L.E. Relative impedance measurements in young children. *Arch. Otolaryngol.,* 1968, *88,* 162-168.
159. Rosenau, H. Die schlafbeschallung: Eine methode der horprufung beim kleinstkind. *Zietschrift fur Laryngol., Rhinol., Otolog. & Ihre Grezgebiete,* 1962, *41,* 194-208.
160. Rosenberg, P., Lovrinic, J., Katinsky, S., & Pikus, A. *Some observations on neonatal hearing screening.* Paper presented at the ASHA Convention, Washington, D.C., 1968.
161. Ross, M., & Lerman, J. Word intelligibility by picture identification (WIPI), Pittsburgh: Stanwix House, 1971.
162. Ruben, R.J. Cochlear potentials as a diagnostic test in deafness. In A.B. Graham (Ed.), *Sensorineural hearing processes and disorders.* Boston: Little, Brown & Co., 1967, pp. 313-337.
163. Ruben, R.J., Bordley, J.E., Nager, G.T., Sekula, J., Knickerbocker, G.G., & Fisch, U. Human cochlear responses to sound stimuli. *Ann. Otol. Rhinol., Laryngol.,* 1960, *169,* 459.
164. Ruben, R.J., Knickerbocker, G.G., Sekula, J., Nayer, G.T., & Bordley, J.E. Cochlear microphonics in man. *Laryngoscope,* 1959, *69,* 665.
165. Ruhn, H.B. Lateral specificity of acoustically evoked EEG responses: 1. Non-verbal, non-meaningful stimuli. *J. Aud. Res.,* 1971, *11,* 1-8.
166. Schulman, C.A., Smith, C.R., Weisinger, M., & Fay, T.H. The use of heart rate in the audiological evaluation of non-verbal children: I. Evaluation of children at risk for hearing impairment. *Neuropaediatrie,* 1970, *2,* 187-196.
167. Schulman, C.A., & Wade, G. The use of heart rate in the audiological evaluation of non-verbal children: II. Clinical trials on an infant population. *Neuropaediatrie,* 1970, *2,* 197-205.
168. Siegenthaler, B., & Haspiel, G. *Development of two standardized measures of hearing for speech by children.* (O.E. Proj. #2372, Contract #OE-5-10-003) 1966.
169. Simmons, F.B., & Russ, F.N. Automated newborn hearing screening, the crib-o-gram. *Arch. Otolaryngol.,* 1974, *100,* 1-7.
170. Speaks, C., & Jerger, J. Method for measurement of speech identification. *J. Speech Hearing Res.,* 1965, *8,* 185-194.
171. Spradlin, J.E., & Lloyd, L.L. Operant conditioning audiometry (OCA) with low level retardates: A preliminary report. In L.L. Lloyd & D.R. Frisina (Eds.), *The audiologic assessment of the mentally retarded: Proceedings of a national conference.* Parsons, Ks.: Speech & Hearing Dept., Parsons State Hosp. Training Cr., 1965, pp. 45-58.
172. Steinschneider, A., Lipton, E.L., & Richmond, J.B. Auditory sensitivity in the infant: Effect of intensity on cardiac and motor responsivity. *Child Develpm.,* 1966, *37,* 233-252.

173. Stewart, J.M. Unpublished report summarized by J.L. Northern & M.P. Downs, *Hearing in children*. Baltimore: Williams & Wilkins, 1974, pp. 111-112.

174. Suzuki, T., & Ogiba, Y. A technique of pure tone audiometry for children under three years of age: Conditioned orientation reflex (C.O.R.) audiometry. *Revue de Laryngol.*, 1960, *1*, 33-45.

175. Tanguay, P.E. A tentative hypothesis concerning the role of hemispheric specialization in early infantile autism. In D.C. Walter (Ed.), *Report of the proceeding of the 1973 conference on cerebral dominance*, Los Angeles: Brain Info. Serv. Publ., 1974, pp. 27-29.

176. Tobias, J. On phonemic analysis of speech discrimination tests. *J. Speech Hearing Res.*, 1964, *7*, 98-100.

177. Thompson, G., & Weber, B.A. Responses of infants and young children to behavior observation audiometry (BOA). *J. Speech Hearing Dis.*, 1974, *39*, 140-147.

178. Trehub, S.E. *Auditory-linguistic sensitivity in infants*. Unpublished doctoral dissertation. McGill University, 1973.

179. Weber, B.A. Validation of observer judgements in behavioral observation audiometry. *J. Speech Hearing Dis.*, 1969, *34*, 350-360.

180. Weber, B.A. Comparison of two approaches to behavioral observation audiometry. *J. Speech Hearing Res.*, 1970, *13*, 823-825.

181. Weber, B.A., & Dybka, M.E. Use of the averaged electroencephalic response in the study of auditory discrimination. *J. Aud. Res.*, 1973, *13*, 45-49.

182. Wedenberg, E. Objective auditory tests on non-cooperative children. *Acta Otolaryngol.*, 1963, (Supplement) *175*, 5-32.

183. Wepman, J. *Auditory discrimination test*. Los Angeles: Western Psychological Services, 1958, (Rev. 1973).

184. Wepman, J. *Auditory Memory Span Test*. Los Angeles: Western Psychological Services, 1973(a).

185. Wepman, J. *Auditory Sequential Memory Test*. Los Angeles: Western Psychological Services, 1973(b).

186. Wever, E.G., & Bray, C.W. Auditory nerve impulses. *Science*, 1930, *71*, 215.

187. Wilson, W.R., & Decker, T.N. *Auditory thresholds of infants using tangible reinforcement operant conditioning audiometry (TROCA) and/or visual reinforcement operant conditioning audiometry (VROCA)*. In preparation.

188. Wilson, W.R., Decker, T.N., Moore, J.M., & Lloyd, L.L. *Behavioral assessment of hearing sensitivity in infants*. Washington, D.C.: Scientific Exhibit, Am. Speech Hearing Assoc. Annual Meeting, 1975.

189. Wilson, W.R., Moore, J.M. & Thompson, G. *Auditory thresholds of infants utilizing visual reinforcement audiometry (VRA)*. In preparation.

190. Withrow, F.B., Jr., & Goldstein, R. An electrophysiologic procedure for determination of auditory threshold in children. *Laryngoscope*, 1958, *68*, 1674-1699.

191. Witkin, B.R., Butler, K.G., Hedrick, D.L., & Manning, C.C. Composite auditory perceptual test (CAPT), Hayward, Ca.: Alameda Cty. School Dept., 1973.

192. Wood, C.C., Goff, W., & Day, R.S. Auditory evoked potentials during speech perception. *Science*, 1971, *173*, 1248-1251.

193. Yarnall, G.D. *Comparison of operant and conventional audiometric procedures with deaf-blind, multiply handicapped children*. Unpublished doctoral dissertation, George Peabody College, 1973.

194. Zeaman, D., & Wegner, N. Cardiac reflex to tone of threshold intensity. *J. Speech Hearing Dis.*, 1956, *21*, 71-75.

Chapter 4

1. Anastasi, A. *Psychological testing* (2nd ed.). New York: Macmillan, 10th printing, 1967.

2. Babbidge Report. *Education of the deaf: A report to the Secretary of Health, Education, and Welfare by his Advisory Committee on the Education of the Deaf*. Washington, D.C.: U.S. Govt. Printing Off., 1965.

3. Battro, A.M. *Piaget: Dictionary of terms*. New York: Pergamon Press, 1973.

4. Becker, S. The performance of deaf and hearing children on a logical discovery task. *Volta Rev.*, 1974, *76*, 537-545.

5. Blank M., & Bridger, W. Conceptual cross-modal transfer in deaf and hearing children. *Child Develpm.*, 1966, *37*, 29-38.

6. Brearley, M., & Hitchfield, E. *A guide to reading Piaget.* New York: Schocken Books, 1969.

7. Brill, R.G. The superior I.Q.'s of deaf children of deaf parents. *California Palms*, Dec. 1969.

134   Bibliography

8. Conrad, R., & Rush, M.L. On the nature of short-term memory encoding by the deaf. *J. Speech Hearing Dis.*, 1965, *30*, 336-343.
9. Crammatte, A.B., (Ed.). *Multiply disabled deaf persons: A manual for rehabilitation counselors.* Washington, D.C.: U.S. Govt. Printing Off., 1970.
10. Cronbach, L.J. *Essentials of psychological testing* (3rd ed.). New York: Harper & Row, 1970.
11. Doehring, D.G., & Rosenstein, J. Speed of visual perception in deaf children. *J. Rehab. Deaf*, 1969, *12*, 118-125.
12. Donoghue, R., & Bolton, B. Psychological evaluation of deaf rehabilitation clients. *J. Rehab. Deaf*, 1971, *5*, 29-38.
13. Elliott, H. Marriage counseling with deaf clients. *J. Rehab. Deaf*, 1974, *8*, 29-35.
14. Falberg, R. The psychological evaluation of prelingually deaf adults. *J. Rehab. Deaf*, 1967, *1*, 31-46.
15. Flavell, J.H. *The developmental psychology of Jean Piaget.* Princeton, N.J.: D. Van Nostrand, 1963.
16. Frey, R.M., & Krause, I.B. The incidence of color blindness among deaf children. *Except. Child.*, 1971, *5*, 393-394.
17. Furth, H.G. *Thinking without language.* New York: Free Press, 1966.
18. Furth, H.G. *Piaget for teachers.* Englewood Cliffs, N.J.: Prentice-Hall, 1970.
19. Furth, H.G. Linguistic deficiency and thinking: Research with deaf subjects 1964-69. *Psychol. Bull.*, 1971, *76*, 58-72.
20. Furth, H.G., & Pufall, P.B. Visual and auditory sequence learning in hearing impaired children. *J. Speech Hearing Res.*, 1966, *9*, 441-449.
21. Furth, H.G., & Youniss, J. Formal operations and language: A comparison of deaf and hearing adolescents. *Internat. J. Psychol.*, 1971, *6*, 49-64.
22. Furth, H.G. & Wachs, H. *Thinking goes to school: Piaget's theory in practice.* New York: Oxford University Press, 1974.
23. Garner, W.R. The acquisition and application of knowledge: A symbiotic relation. *Am. Psychol.*, 1972, *27*, 941-946.
24. Garrett, J.F., & Levine, E.S. *Rehabilitation practices with the physically disabled.* New York: Columbia University Press, 1973.
25. Giangreco, C.J. The Hiskey-Nebraska Test of Learning Aptitude (Rev.) compared to several achievement tests. *Am. Ann. Deaf*, 1966, *111*, 566-577.
26. Gilbert, J.G., & Levee, R.F. Performance of deaf and normally hearing children on the Bender-Gestalt and the Archimedes Spiral Tests. *Percept. Motor Skills*, 1967, *24*, 1059-1066.
27. Goetzinger, C.P. Factors associated with counseling the hearing impaired adult. *J. Rehab. Deaf*, 1967, *1*, 32-48.
28. Goetzinger, C.P., Ortiz, J.D., Bellerose, B., & Buchan, L.G. A study of the S.O. Rroschach with deaf and hearing adolescents. *Am. Ann. Deaf*, 1966, *3*, 510-522.
29. Goetzinger, C.P., Wills, R.C., & Dekker, L.C. Non-language I.Q. tests used with deaf pupils. *Volta Rev.*, 1967, *69*, 500-506.
30. Goetzinger, M.R., & Houchins, R.R. The 1947 Colored Raven's Progressive Matrices with deaf and hearing subjects. *Am. Ann. Deaf*, 1969, *114*, 95-101.
31. Hoemann, H.W., Andrews, C.E., & deRosa, D.V. Categorical encoding in short-term memory by deaf and hearing children. *J. Speech Hearing Res.* 1974, *17*, 426-431.
32. Hurder, W.P. Research on the hearing impaired. In UNESCO, *The present situation and trends of research in the field of special education.* Paris, 1973.
33. Kates, S.L. The categorization of simulated love and anger scenes by deaf and hearing adults. In S.L. Kates, *Cognitive structures in deaf, hearing, and psychotic individuals.* Northampton, Ma.: The Clarke School for the Deaf, 1967.
34. Kates, S.L. Learning and use of logical symbols by deaf and hearing subjects. *J. Abnorm. Psychol.*, 1969, *74*, 699-705.
35. Kates, S.L. *Language development in deaf and hearing adolescents.* Northampton, Ma.: The Clarke School for the Deaf, 1972.
36. Kearney, J.E. A new performance scale of cognitive capacity for use with deaf subjects. *Am. Ann. Deaf*, 1969, *114*, 2-14.
37. Keogh, B.K., Vernon, M., & Smith, C.E. Deafness and visuo-motor function. *J. Spec. Educ.*, 1970, *4*, 41-47.
38. Lane, H.S., & Baker, D. Reading achievement of the deaf: Another look. *Volta Rev.*, 1974, *76*, 489-499.
39. Lantz, D., & Lenneberg, E.M. Verbal communication and color memory in deaf and hearing. *Child Develpm.*, 1966, *37*, 765-779.

40. Lawson, L., Jr., & Myklebust, H. Opthalmological deficiencies in deaf children. *Except. Child.*, 1970, *37*, 17-20.
41. Lennan, R.K. The deaf multi-handicapped unit at the California School for the Deaf, Riverside. *Am. Ann. Deaf*, 1973, *118*, 439-445.
42. Levine, E.S. *Youth in a soundless world.* New York: University Press, 1956.
43. Levine, E.S. Studies in psychological evaluation of the deaf. *Volta Rev.*, 1963, *65*, 496-512. (Special issue research)
44. Levine, E.S. Mental assessment of the deaf child. *Volta Rev.*, 1971, *73*, 80-96, 97-105.
45. Levine, E.S. *Lisa and her soundless world.* New York: Behavioral Publications, 1974(a).
46. Levine, E.S. Psychological tests and practices with the deaf: A survey of the state of the art. *Volta Rev.*, 1974b, *76*, 298-319.
47. Levine, E.S. Psychological evaluation of the deaf client. In B. Bolton (Ed.), *Handbook of measurement and evaluation in rehabilitation.* Baltimore: University Park Press, in press.
48. Levine, E.S., & Naiman, D. (Eds.), Seminar on behavior modification for psychologists working with the deaf. *Am. Ann. Deaf*, 1970, *115*, 455-491. (Special issue)
49. Levine, E.S., & Wagner, E.E. Personality patterns of deaf persons: An interpretation based on research with the Hand Test. *Percept. Motor Skills*, 1974, (Monogr. Suppl. 4-V39)
50. Michael, J., & Kates, S.L. Concept attainment on social materials by deaf and hearing adolescents. *J. Educ. Psychol.*, 1965, *56*, 81-86.
51. Meadow, K.P. Early manual communication in relation to the deaf child's intellectual, social, and communicative functioning. *Am. Ann. Deaf*, 1968, *113*, 29-41.
52. Musgrove, W.J., & Counts, L. Leiter and Raven performance and teacher ranking: A correlation study with deaf children. *J. Rehab. Deaf*, 1975, *8*, 18-22.
53. Nix, G.W. Total communication: A review of the studies offered in its support. *Volta Rev.*, 1975, *11*, 470-494.
54. Owrid, H. Studies in manual communication with hearing impaired children. *Volta Rev.*, 1971, *73*, 428-438.
55. Phillips, J.L., Jr., *The origins of intellect Piaget's theory.* San Francisco: W. H. Freeman, 1969.
56. Poulos, T.H. *Attitudes toward the deaf: A Guttman facet theory analysis of their content.* (Doctoral dissertation) Ann Arbor: Michigan State University, 1970, (University Microfilm No. 71-11, 946)
57. Quigley, S.P. *The influence of fingerspelling on the development of language, communication and educational achievement in deaf children.* Urbana, Il.: Inst. Res. Except. Child., 1969.
58. Quigley, S. *Development and description of syntactic structures in the language of deaf children, 1969-1973* (USOE GO-9-232175-4370). Urbana. University of Illinois, Inst Res Except. Child., 1972.
59. Riopelle, A.J. (Ed.). *Animal problem solving.* Baltimore: Penquin Books, 1967.
60. Rister, A. Deaf children in mainstream education. *Volta Rev.*, 1975, *77*, 279-290.
61. Robertson, A., & Youniss, J. Anticipatory visual imagery in deaf and hearing children. *Child Develpm.*, 1969, *40*, 123-135.
62. Ross, B.M. Probability concepts in deaf and hearing children. *Child Develpm.*, 1966, *37*, 917-927.
63. Ross, D.R. A technique of verbal ability assessment of deaf adults. *J. Rehab. Deaf*, 1970, *3*, 7-15.
64. Sanders, J.W., & Coscarelli, J.E. The relationship of visual synthesis skill to lipreading. *Volta Rev.*, 1970, *115*, 23-26.
65. Schiff, W. Social perception in deaf and hearing adolescents. *Except. Child.*, 1973, *39*, 289-297.
66. Schiff, W., & Dytell, R.S. Deaf and hearing children's performance on a tactual perception battery. *Percept. Motor Skills.* 1972. (Monogr. Suppl. 2-V35)
67. Schiff, S., & Saxe, E. Person perceptions of deaf and hearing observers viewing filmed interactions. *Percept. Motor Skills*, 1972, *35*, 219-234.
68. Schiff, W., & Thayer, S. An eye for an ear? Social perception, nonverbal communication and deafness. *Rehab. Psychol.*, 1974, *21*, 50-70.
69. Schlesinger, H., & Meadow, K.P. *Sound and sign.* Berkeley: California University Press, 1972.
70. Siebert, W.F., & Snow, R.E. Cine-psychometry. *AV Communic. Rev.*, 1965, *13*, 140-158.
71. Stevens, W.D. Affection and cognition in transaction and the mapping of cultural space. *AV Communic. Rev.*, 1970, *18*, 440-445.
72. Stevenson, E.A. A study of the educational achievement of deaf children of deaf parents. *Maryland Bull.*, Feb. 1965, pp. 63-64; 69; 74.

73. Stewart, L.G. Problems of severely handicapped deaf. *Am. Ann. Deaf,* 1971, *116,* 362-368.
74. Stuckless, E.R., & Birch, J.W. The influence of early manual communication on the linguistic development of deaf children. *Am. Ann. Deaf,* 1966, *111,* 452-460.
75. Suchman, R.G. Color-form preference, discriminative accuracy and learning of deaf and hearing children. *Child Develpm.,* 1966, *37,* 439-451.
76. Sussman, A.E., & Stewart, L.G. (Eds.). *Counseling with deaf people.* New York: University Deafness Res. Training Cr., 1971.
77. Vegely, A.B. Performance of hearing-impaired children on a nonverbal personality test. *Am. Ann. Deaf,* 1971, *116,* 427-434.
78. Vegely, A.B., & Elliott, L.L. Applicability of standardized personality test to a hearing-impaired population. *Am. Ann. Deaf,* 1968, *113,* 858-869.
79. Vernon, M. Psychological evaluation of the hearing impaired for the job corps. *Proceedings of the National Conference on the Feasibility of Integrating Deaf Youth into the Job Corps.* Washington, D.C.: Off. Econ. Opport., 1965.
80. Vernon, M. Failure of education of the deaf. *State Wide Bull. Illinois Assoc. Deaf,* 1967, *5,* 8-15.
81. Vernon, M. Fifty years of research on the intelligence of the deaf and hard-of-hearing, *J. Rehab. Deaf,* 1968, *2,* 1-12.
82. Vernon, M. *Multiply handicapped deaf children: Medical, educational, and psychological considerations.* Washington, D.C.: Coun. Except. Child., 1969a.
83. Vernon, M. Techniques of screening for mental illness in deaf clients. *J. Rehab. Deaf,* 1969b, *2,* 22-36.
84. Vernon, M., & Koh, S.D. Early manual communication and deaf children's achievement. *Am. Ann. Deaf,* 1969, *115,* 529-536.
85. Vernon, M. & Koh, S.D. Effects of oral preschool compared to early manual communication on education and communication in deaf children. *Am. Ann. Deaf,* 1970, *116,* 569-574.
86. Withrow, F.B. Immediate memory span of deaf and normally hearing children, *Except. Child.,* 1968, *35,* 33-41.
87. Wrightstone, J., Aronow, M., & Moskowitz, S. Developing reading test norms for deaf children. *Am. Ann. Deaf,* 1963, *108,* 311-316.
88. Youniss, J., & Furth, H.G. The influence of transitivity on learning in hearing and deaf children. *Child Develpm.,* 1965, *36,* 533-538.
89. Youniss, J., Furth, H.G., & Ross, B.M. Logical symbol use in deaf and hearing children and adolescents. *Develpm. Psychol.,* 1971, *3,* 511-517.
90. Zivkovic, M. Influence of deafness on the structure of personality. *Percept. Motor Skills,* 1971, *33,* 863-866.

Chapter 5

1. Adler, E.P. (Ed.). *Deafness.* Silver Spring, Md.: Prof. Rehab. Workers with Adult Deaf, 1969, Monograph No. 1.
2. Altshuler, D. *A unique innovation in the development of a comprehensive vocational rehabilitation facility for the deaf* (Final Report Project no. X29-67). May, 1971. (Mimeographed)
3. Boatner, E.B., Stuckless, E.R., & Moore, D.F. *Occupational status of the young adult deaf of New England and demand for a regional technical-vocational training center.* West Hartford, Ct.: American School for the Deaf, 1964.
4. Bowe, F., & Watson, D. A new approach to serving deaf people. *Soc. Rehab. Rec.,* Dec. 1974-Jan. 1975, *2,* 1, 11-14.
5. Bowe, F., & Watson, D. Rehabilitation with deaf people: Four models for facilitating service delivery. *Rehab. Lit.,* 1975, *36,* 44-47.
6. Bowe, F., Watson, D., & Anderson, G. Delivery of community services to deaf persons. *J. Rehab. Deaf,* 1973, *7,* 1, 15-29.
7. Blake, G. Services for deaf adults at Hot Springs Rehabilitation Center. *J. Rehab. Deaf,* 1968, *2,* 1, 28-31.
8. Brookey, J.M. The Seattle Community College, new program for deaf people. *J. Rehab. Deaf,* 1969, *3,* 1, 52-60.
9. Coleman, T.J., Ethridge, W.A., Atelsek, F.J., & Meisegeier, R. *Serving deaf adults: Development of innovative patterns of community services for the adult deaf.* Silver Spring, Md.: Nat. Assoc. of Hearing and Speech Agencies, 1973.
10. Craig, W.N., & Silver, N.J. Examination of selected employment problems of the deaf. *Am. Ann. Deaf,* 1966, *111,* 544-549.

11. Crammatte, A.B. *Deaf persons in professional employment*. Springfield, Il.: Charles C Thomas, 1968.
12. Crammatte, A.B., & Miles, D.S. (Eds.). *Multiply disabled deaf persons: A manual for rehabilitation counselers* (SRS 73-25047). Washington, D.C.: U.S. Dept. HEW, 1968.
13. Culton, P.M. (Ed.). *Operation TRIPOD* (HEW RSA Grant No. 44-P-45085/9-10). Washington, D.C.: U.S. Dept. HEW, April 1971.
14. Ethridge, W.A. Community referral services. *J. Rehab. Deaf*, 1969, *3*, 1, 103-111.
15. Frisina, D.R. NTID and higher education for deaf persons. *J. Rehab. Deaf*, 1969, *3*, 1, 28-33.
16. Gellman, W. Projections in the field of physical disability. *Rehab. Lit*, 1974, *35*, 1, 2-9.
17. Garretson, M.D. Introduction, In H.G. Kopp (Ed.), *Accent on unity: Horizons on deafness*. Washington, D.C.: Counc. Org. Serv. Deaf, April 1968, p. 9.
18. Hairston, E.E. Diagnostic evaluation and adjustment facility (Project D.E.A.F.). *J. Rehab. Deaf*, 1971, *5*, 1, 24-38.
19. Hurwitz, S.D. *Habilitation of deaf young adults* (HEW SRS Final Report no. RD-1804-S). St. Louis: Jewish Employment and Vocational Service, 1971.
20. Kronenberg, H.H., & Blake, G.D. *Young deaf adults: An occupational survey*. Washington, D.C.: Vocational Rehabilitation Administration, 1966.
21. Lauritsen, R.R. President's address - Trends in PRWAD. *J. Rehab. Deaf*, 1971, *4*, 3, 16-22.
22. Lawrence, C.A., & Vescove, G.M. *Deaf adults in New England: An exploratory service program* (HEW SRS Final Report no. RD- 1516-S). Boston: Morgan Memorial Hospital, 1967.
23. Lloyd, G.T. *State coordinators of the deaf workshop*. Silver Spring, Md.: Prof. Rehab. Workers with Adult Deaf, in press.
24. Lunde, A.A., & Bigman, S.K. *Occupational conditions among the deaf*. Washington, D.C.: Gallaudet College, 1959.
25. Nelson, C.D. *The St. Paul Technical Institute Program for deaf students*. *J. Rehab. Deaf*, 1969, *3*, 1, 61-68.
26. Peterson, E. Crossroads Rehabilitation Center Program for the Deaf. *J. Rehab. Deaf*, 1974, *8*, 1, 29-32.
27. Pimentel, A.T. Interpreting services for deaf people. *J. Rehab. Deaf*, 1969, *3*, 1, 112-119.
28. Quigley, S.P. (Ed.). *The vocational rehabilitation of deaf people*. Washington, D.C.: U.S. Dept. HEW, 1966.
29. Rainer, J.D., Altshuler, K.A., Kallman, F.J., & Deming, W.E. (Eds.). *Family and mental health problems in a deaf population*. New York: New York State Psychiatric Inst., Dept. Med. Gen., 1963.
30. Rawlings, D.W., Trybus, R.J., Delgado, G.I. & Stuckless, E.R. *A guide to college career programs for deaf students* (Rev. ed.). Gallaudet College & NTID, Sept. 1975.
31. Reece, O.E. *Inventory on services for rehabilitation of deaf clients - Implementation of model state plan*. Jan. 1976. (Mimeographed)
32. Rice, B.D. *A comprehensive facility program for multiply handicapped deaf adults* (HEW SRS Final Report Project no. 14-p-55216, Grant no. 16-P-56812, RT-13). Fayetteville: Arkansas Rehabilitation Research and Training Ctr., May 1973.
33. Romano, Frank. Interpreter consortium: A sign for the future. *Soc. Rehab. Rec.* Dec. 1974 - Jan. 1975, *2*, 1, 10.
34. Schein, J.D. *The deaf community: Studies of the social phychology of deafness*. Washington, D.C.: Gallaudet Press, 1968.
35. Schein, J.D. (Ed.). Model for a state plan for vocational rehabilitation of deaf clients. Silver Spring, Md.: Prof. Rehab. Workers with Adult Deaf, 1973, Monograph No. 3.
36. Schein, J.D., & Bushnag, S.M. Higher education for the deaf in the United States: A retrospective investigation. *Am. Ann. Deaf*, 1962, *107*, 416-420.
37. Schein, J.D., & Delk, M.T. *The deaf population of the United States*. Silver Spring, Md.: Nat. Assoc. Deaf, 1974.
38. Smith, J. Open letter to officers of PRWAD and RID. *Deaf Am*, 1975, *28*, 3, p. 29.
39. Smith, J.M. (Ed.). *Workshop on interpreting for the deaf*, Muncie, In.: Ball State Teachers College, 1964.
40. Stewart, L.G. Problems of severely handicapped deaf: Implications for educational programs. *Am. Ann. Deaf*, 1971, *116*, 362-368.
41. Stewart, L.G., & Schein, J.D. *Tarrytown Conference on Current Priorities in the Rehabilitation of Deaf People*. New York: New York Deafness Research & Training Center, 1971.
42. Vernon, M. Potential achievement and rehabilitation in the deaf population. *Rehab. Lit.*, 1970, *31*, 9, 258-267.
43. Watson, D. Improving rehabilitation service delivery for severely handicapped deaf persons through research utilization. *J. Rehab. Deaf*, 1974, *8*, 1, 85-86.

44. Watson, D. Improving service delivery to deaf inner city residents. *Proceedings of the VII Congress of the World Federation of the Deaf.* Washington, D.C.: Nat. Assoc. Deaf, in press.
45. Watson, D., Bowe, F.G., & Schein, J.D. *Orientation to deafness: A curriculum guide.* New York: New York University, Deafness Research & Training Ctr, 1973. (Mimeographed)
46. Watson, D., & Stemberg, M. *Guidelines for vocational evaluation of deaf and hearing impaired clients.* New York: New York University, Deafness Research & Training Ctr., (In preparation)
47. Wells, D.O. The Delgado College Academic & Vocational Education Program for the Deaf. *J. Rehab. Deaf,* 1969, *3,* 1, 44-51.
48. Woodrick, W.E., Scalf, L.C., & Lloyd, G.T. Training needs of rehabilitative personnel serving deaf persons. *Deafness Ann.,* 1974, *4,* 45-54.

Chapter 6

1. Morkovin, B.V. Experiment in teaching deaf preschool children in the Soviet Union. *Volta Rev.,* 1960, *62,* 260-268.

Chapter 7

1. Bjorlee, I. *Proceedings of the Twenty-Seventh Meeting, Conference of Executives of American Schools for the Deaf.* Washington, D.C.: Am. Ann. Deaf, 1955, pp. 302-304; 323.
2. Bjorlee, I. Report of the chairman of the conference executive committee. *Am. Ann. Deaf,* 1949, *94,* 167-175.
3. Bjorlee, I., & Brill, R.G. Report of the committee on teacher training and certification. *Proceedings of the Twenty-Third Meeting, Conference of Executives of American Schools for the Deaf,* Washington, D.C.: Am. Ann. Deaf, 1951, pp. 172-175.
4. Brill, R.G. Report of the committee on teacher training and certification. *Am. Ann. Deaf,* 1951, *96,* 407-409.
5. Brill, R.G. Report on the council on education of the deaf. *Proceedings of the Fortieth Meeting, Conference of Executives of American Schools for the Deaf,* Washington, D.C.: Am. Ann. Deaf, 1968, pp. 122-123.
6. Farrar, A. *Arnold on the education of the deaf.* London: Nat. Coll. Teachers Deaf, 1923, pp. 93-102.
7. French, S.L. Reflections on twenty years of preparation of teachers of deaf children. *Proceedings of the Forty-Fifth Meeting of the Conference, Executives of American Schools for the Deaf.* Washington, D.C.: Am. Ann. Deaf, 1971, pp. 619-624.
8. Fusfeld, I.S. A teacher training center in California. *Am. Ann. Deaf,* 1934, *79,* pp. 88-89.
9. Fusfeld, I.S. Certification requirements and report on certification of teachers. *Am. Ann. Deaf,* 1932, *77,* 3-11.
10. Hall, P. Report of the chairman of the executive committee of the Conference of Executives of American Schools for the Deaf. *Am. Ann. Deaf,* 1932, *77,* 1-2.
11. Hall, P. Report of the executive committee of the conference. *Am. Ann. Deaf,* 1933, *78,* 349-352.
12. Hall, P., & Bjorlee, I. A plan for the certification of teachers (Conference Proceedings). *Am. Ann. Deaf,* 1931, *76,* 153-159; 331-334.
13. Hoag, R.L. Proposed standards for the certification of teachers of the hearing impaired. *Proceedings of the Forty-Third Meeting, Conference of Executives of American Schools for the Deaf.* Washington, D.C.: Am. Ann. Deaf, 1971, pp. 747-758.
14. Hoag, R.L. Standards for the certification of teachers of the hearing impaired. *Proceedings of the Conference of Executives of American Schools for the Deaf,* Washington, D.C.: Am. Ann. Deaf, 1973, pp. 756-761.
15. Hoffmeyer, B.E. Report of council on education of the deaf. *Proceedings of the Forty-Third Meeting, Conference of Executives of American Schools for the Deaf,* Washington, D.C.: Am. Ann. Deaf, 1971, p. 747.
16. Jones, J.W., Pittinger, O.M., & Taylor, H. The training and certification of teachers (Proceedings of the Fourteenth Conference of Superintendents and Principals of American Schools for the Deaf). *Am. Ann. Deaf,* 1929, *74,* 245-251.
17. Long, J.S. The certification of teachers. *Am. Ann. Deaf,* 1931, *76,* 378-392.

18. Mackie, R.P., & Dunn, L.M. State certification requirements for teachers of exceptional children. *Bulletin,* 1954, no. 1, Washington, D.C.: U.S. Office of Education, HEW.
19. Mangan, K.R. Report of the joint committee on teacher training and certification. *Proceedings of the Forty-First Meeting, Conference of Executives of the American Schools for the Deaf,* Washington, D.C.: Am. Ann. Deaf, 1969, pp. 560-561.
20. Moore, L.M. Report of the joint committee on teacher training and certification. *Proceedings of the Thirty-Ninth Meeting, Conference of Executives of the American Schools for the Deaf,* Washington, D.C.: Am. Ann. Deaf, 1967, pp. 40-41.
21. Preparation of teachers of the deaf (Nat. Conf. Report, Virginia Beach, Va., 1964 - OE-35059) *Bulletin,* 1966, no. 8, Washington, D.C.: U.S. Office of Educ., HEW.
22. *Proceedings of the Forty-First Meeting, Conference of Executives of the American Schools for the Deaf.* Washington, D.C.: *Am. Ann. Deaf,* 1969, pp. 514-528.
23. *Proceedings of the Thirty-Seventh Meeting, Conference of Executives,* Washington, D.C.: *Am. Ann. Deaf,* 1965, pp. 525-528.
24. *Proceedings of the Twenty-First Conference,* Washington, D.C.: *Am. Ann. Deaf,* 1949, pp. 163-165.
25. Quigley, H.M., & Stelle, R.M. *Proceedings of the Thirty-Eighth Meeting, Conference of Executives of the American Schools for the Deaf,* Washington, D.C.: *Am. Ann. Deaf,* 1966, pp. 104-114.
26. Silverman, S.R. *Conference summary and impressions: Education of the deaf—The challenge and the charge.* (Report of the Nat. Conf. Educ. Deaf, Colorado Springs, Co.). 1967, pp. 137-142.
27. Stelle, R.M. Report of teacher training and certification committee. *Proceedings of the Thirty-Ninth Meeting, Conference of Executives of the American Schools for the Deaf,* Washington, D.C.: *Am. Ann. Deaf,* 1967, pp. 461-464.
28. Taylor, H. Raising standards of teacher training. *Am. Ann. Deaf,* 1934, 79, 185.
29. Yale, C., & Committee. Report of the committee on standardization of normal courses for teachers of the deaf. Am. Ann. Deaf, 1927, 72, 153-159.

Chapter 8

1. Craig, W.N. (Ed.). *Directory of programs and services.* Washington, D.C.: Am. Ann. Deaf, 1974, 1975.
2. Craig, W.N., Craig, H.B., & Burke, R. Components of verbotonal instruction for deaf students. *Lang., Speech Hearing Schools,* 1974, 5, 38-43.
3. Craig, H.B., & Holman, G.L. The open classroom in a school for the deaf. *Am. Ann. Deaf,* 1973, 118, 675-685.
4. Craig, W.N., & Salem, J. Partial integration of deaf with hearing students. *Am. Ann. Deaf,* 1975, 120, 28-36.
5. *Curriculum for underachieving deaf students* and *Consumer education curriculum guide* (Reports). St. Augustine: Florida School for Deaf and Blind, 1974.
6. Grammatico, L.F., & Miller, S.D. Curriculum for the preschool deaf child. *Volta Rev.,* 1974, 74, 280-289.
7. *Health sciences; Cooperative education; Daily living skills* (Reports). Jacksonville: Illinois School for Deaf, 1965-1975.
8. Keith, J.B., & Gluck, M.R. Profile of diagnostic information designed to describe the individual learner. *Peabody J. Educ.,* 1974. (reprint from Colliers Speech & Hearing Cr.)
9. Lennan, R.K. The multi-handicapped unit at the California School for the Deaf, Riverside. *Am. Ann. Deaf,* 1974, 118, 439-445.
10. McCarr, D. *Materials used for deaf hearing impaired.* Lake Oswego, Or.: Dormac, 1975.
11. Pfau, G.S. *Instructional manual for the general electric, Project LIFE program.* Ballston Lake, N.Y.: Industrial Industries, 1974.
12. Schein, J.D. Deaf students with other disabilities. *Am. Ann. Deaf,* 1975, 120, 92-99.
13. Stepp, R.E. Personal correspondence dated October 6, 1975 in response to a request for curriculum information.
14. Trybus, R.J. (and previously Ries, P.) *Annual survey of hearing impaired children and youth.* Washington, D.C.: Gallaudet College, ODS, 1968-1975.
15. Uno, A.O. *Aesthetic activities for handicapped children.* Austin, Tx: Texas Educ. Agency, 1973.
16. Wolff, S., & Wolff, C. *Games without words.* Springfield, Ill.: Charles C Thomas, 1974.

Chapter 8   Selected References

The following selected references, not previously cited, may be of interest to schools planning changes in curriculum.

1. Clarke School for the Deaf. *Lower school five year curriculum guide* (Report). Northampton, Ma., 1974.
2. Colorado School for the Deaf and the Blind. *Curriculum outline* (Report). Colorado Springs, 1974.
3. Lexington School for the Deaf. *Education series* (9 vols.) (Report). New York, 1960-1974.
4. Marie H. Katzenbach School for the Deaf. *Publications for use with deaf students* (Report). West Trenton, N.J., 1965-1975.
5. New Mexico School for the Deaf. *Preschool curriculum giude* (Report). Albuquerque, 1975. (mimeographed)
6. Rhode Island School for the Deaf. *The language curriculum* (Report). Providence, 1971.
7. Craig, H.B., Craig, W.N., Bram, P., & Neisworth, R. *Evaluation manual* (Report). Pittsburgh: Western Pennsylvania School for the Deaf, 1974.
8. Craig, W., & Collins, J. Communication patterns of deaf students. *Except. Child.*, 1970, 37, 283-289.
9. Furth, H., & Wachs, H. *Thinking goes to school.* New York: Oxford Press, 1975.
10. Gantenbein, A.R. *Preschool curriculum* (Report). Berrien Springs, Mi.: Berrien Cty. Day Prog. for Hearing Impaired Child., 1975.
11. Harrington, J. D. The integration of deaf children and youth through education strategies. *Highlights*, 1974, 53, (reprint from N.Y. League for Hard of Hrg.)
12. Hicks, D. E., & Ferguson, D. G. *Secondary education for the deaf* (Report). Washington, D.C.: Gallaudet College, 1975.
13. Kopp, H.G. Curriculum: Cognition and content. *Volta Rev.*, 1968, 70, #6. (Monograph)
14. Lorene, S.J. *The what, when, and how of teaching language to deaf children.* St. Louis, Missouri: Fontbonne College, 1968.
15. Peck, B.J. *Patterned languagc program* (Report). Salem: Oregon State School for the Deaf, 1974.
16. Restaino, L.C. *Curriculum for young deaf children.* Albany, N.Y.: State Educ, Dept., 1971.
17. Stepp, R. Symposium on research and utilization of educational media for teaching the deaf. *Am. Ann. Deaf*, 1965-1974, 110-119. (Fall issues)

Chapter 9

1. Bach, E., & Harms, R. *Universals in linguistic theory.* New York: Holt, Rinehart, & Winston, 1968.
2. Bellugi, U., & Klima, E. Aspects of sign language and its structure. In J. Kavanagh & J. Cutting (Eds.), *The role of speech in language.* Cambridge: MIT Press, 1975, 171-203.
3. Bellugi, U., Klima, E., & Siple, P. Remembering in signs. *Cognition*, 1974, 3, 93-125.
4. Berko-Gleason, J. The child's learning of English morphology. *Word*, 1958, 14, 150-177.
5. Bever, T. The cognitive basis for linguistic structures. In J. Hayes (Ed.), *Cognition and the development of language.* New York: Wiley, 1970, pp. 279-352.
6. Bloom, L. *Language development: Form and function in emerging grammars.* Cambridge: MIT Press, 1970.
7. Bloom, L. Why not pivot grammar? *J. Speech Hearing Dis.*, 1971, 36, 40-51.
8. Bloom, L. *One word at a time: The use of single word utterances before syntax.* The Hague: Mouton, 1973.
9. Bloom, L., Hood, L., & Lightbrown, P. Imitation in language development: If, when and why. *Cog. Psychol.*, 1974, 6, 380-420.
10. Bowerman, M. *Early syntactic development: A cross-linguistic study with special reference to Finnish.* Cambridge: Cambridge University Press, 1973.
11. Braine, M. The ontogeny of English phrase structure: The first phase. *Language*, 1963, 39, 1-13.
12. Brown, R. *A first language: The early stages.* Cambridge: Harvard University Press, 1973.
13. Brown, R., & Fraser, C. The acquisition of syntax. In U. Bellugi & R. Brown (Eds.), *The acquisition of language.* Lafayette: Monogr. Soc. Res. Child Develpm., 1964, 43-79.
14. Chafe, W. *Meaning and the structure of language.* Chicago: University of Chicago Press, 1970.
15. Chomsky, C. *The acquisition of syntax in children from 5 to 10.* Cambridge: MIT Press, 1969.

16. Chomsky, N. *Syntactic structures*. The Hague: Mouton, 1957.
17. Chomsky, N. *Aspects of the theory of syntax*. Cambridge: MIT Press, 1965.
18. Chomsky, N. *Language and mind*. New York: Harcourt, Brace, Jovanovich, 1972.
19. Clark, E. How children describe time and order. In C. Ferguson & D. Slobin (Eds.), *Studies of child language development*. New York: Holt, Rinehart, & Winston, 1973a, pp. 585-606.
20. Clark, E. Non-linguistic strategies and the acquisition of word meanings. *Cognition*, 1973b, *2*, 161-182.
21. Cooper, R. The ability of deaf and hearing children to apply morphological rules. *J. Speech Hearing Res.*, 1967, *10*, 77-86.
22. Cooper, R., & Rosenstein, J. Language acquisition of deaf children. *Volta Rev.*, 1966, *68*, 46-56.
23. De Villiers, P., & De Villiers, J. Early judgements of semantic and syntactic acceptability by children. *J. Psycholing. Res.*, 1972, *1*, 299-310.
24. Donaldson, M., & Balfour, G. Less is more: A study of language comprehension in children. *Brit. J. Psychol.*, 1968, *59*, 461-472.
25. Donaldson, M., & Wales, R. On the acquisition of some relational terms. In J. Hayes (Ed.), *Cognition and the development of language*. New York: Wiley, 1970, pp. 235-268.
26. Eimas, P. Linguistic processing of speech by young infants. In R. Schiefelbusch, & L. Lloyd (Eds.), *Language perspectives - Acquisition, retardation, and intervention*. Baltimore: University Park Press, 1974.
27. Eisenberg, R. *Auditory competence in early life*. Baltimore: University Park Press, 1975.
28. Ervin-Tripp, S. Discourse agreement: How children answer questions. In J. Hayes (Ed.), *Cognition and the development of language*. New York: Wiley, 1970, pp. 95-107.
29. Ervin-Tripp, S. Social backgrounds and verbal skills. In R. Huxley, & E. Ingram (Eds.), *Language acquisition: Models and methods*. New York: Academic Press, 1971, pp. 29-37.
30. Filmore, C., & Langendoen, D. *Studies in linguistic semantics*. New York: Holt, Rinehart, & Winston, 1971.
31. Fishman, J. *Advances in the sociology of language*. The Hague: Mouton, 1972.
32. Hess, L. *A longitudinal transformational generative comparison of the emerging syntactic structures in a deaf child and a normally hearing child* Unpublished master thesis. University of Cincinnati, 1972.
33. Huttenlocher, J. The origins of language comprehension. In R. Solso (Ed.), *Theories in cognitive psychology: The Loyola Symposium*. New York: Wiley, 1974, pp. 331-368.
34. Huttenlocher, J. Encoding information in sign language. In J. Kavanagh, & J. Cutting (Eds.), *The role of speech in language*. Cambridge: MIT Press, 1975, pp. 229-239.
35. Huttenlocher, J., Eisenberg, K., & Strauss, S. Comprehension: Relation between perceived actor and logical subject. *J. Verb. Learn. Verb. Behav.*, 1968, *7*, 527-530.
36. Hymes, D. Competence and performance in linguistic theory. In R. Huxley, & E. Ingram (Eds.), *Language acquisition: Models and methods*. New York: Academic Press, 1971, pp. 2-34.
37. Ingram, D. The relationship between comprehension and production. In R. Schiefelbusch, & L. Lloyd (Eds.), *Language perspectives - Acquisition, retardation, and intervention*. Baltimore: University Park Press, 1974, pp. 313-334.
38. Jackendorff, R. *Semantic interpretation in generative grammar*. Cambridge: MIT Press, 1972.
39. Katz, J. *Semantic theory*. New York: Harper & Row, 1972.
40. Klima, E., & Bellugi, U. The roots of language in the sign talk of the deaf. *Psychol. Today*, 1972, *6*, 61-64.
41. Kretschmer, R. *Transformational linguistic analysis of the written language of hearing impaired and normal hearing students*. Unpublished doctoral dissertation. Teachers Coll., Columbia University, 1972.
42. Kretschmer, R. *The written language of hearing impaired children: Delayed, deviant or dialect?* Paper presented at ASHA Convention, Washington, D.C., 1975.
43. Limber, J. The genesis of complex sentences. In T. Moore (Ed.), *Cognitive development and the acquisition of language*. New York: Academic Press, 1973, pp. 169-185.
44. McNeill, D. *The acquisition of language: The study of developmental psycholinguistics*. New York: Harper & Row, 1970.
45. Menyuk, P. *Sentences children use*. Cambridge: MIT Press, 1969.
46. Miller, W., & Ervin, S. The development of grammar in child language. In U. Bellugi, & R. Brown (Eds.), *The acquisition of language*. Lafayette: Monogr. Soc. Res. Child Develpm., 1964, pp. 9-34.

47. Morehead, D., & Morehead, A. From signal to sign: A Piagetian view of thought and language during the first two years. In R. Schiefelbusch, & L. Lloyd (Eds.), *Language perspectives - Acquisition, retardation, and intervention.* Baltimore: University Park Press, 1974, pp. 153-190.
48. Morse, P. Infant speech perception: A preliminary model and review of the literature. In R. Schiefelbusch, & L. Lloyd (Eds.), *Language perspectives - Acquisition, retardation, and intervention.* Baltimore: University Park Press, 1974, pp. 17-53.
49. Nelson, K. *Presyntactical strategies for learning to talk.* Paper presented at Soc. for Res. in Child Develpm., Minneapolis, 1971.
50. Power, D., & Quigley, S. Deaf children's acquisition of passive voice. *J. Speech Hearing Res.,* 1973, *16,* 5-11.
51. Quigley, S., Smith, S., & Wilbur, R. Comprehension of relativized sentences by deaf students. *J. Speech Hearing Res.,* 1974, *17,* 325-341.
52. Quigley, S., Wilbur, R., & Montanelli, D. Development of question-formation in the written language of deaf students. *J. Speech Hearing Res.,* 1974, *17,* 699-713.
53. Schiefelbusch, R., & Lloyd, L (Eds.), *Language perspectives - Acquisition, retardation, and intervention.* Baltimore: University Park Press, 1974.
54. Schlesinger, I. The production of utterances and language acquisition. In D. Slobin (Ed.), *The ontogenesis of grammar.* New York: Academic Press, 1971, pp. 63-101.
55. Schmitt, P. *Deaf children's comprehension and production of sentence transformations and verb tenses.* Unpublished doctoral dissertation. University of Illinois, 1968.
56. Sinclair, H. Language acquisition and cognitive development. In T. Moore (Ed.), *Cognitive development and the acquisition of language.* New York: Academic Press, 1973.
57. Slobin, D. Cognitive prerequisites for the development of grammar. In C. Ferguson & D. Slobin (Eds.), *Studies in child language development.* New York: Holt, Rinehart, & Winston, 1973, pp. 175-208.
58. Smith, F. *Comprehension and learning.* New York: Holt, Rinehart, & Winston, 1975.
59. Stokoe, W., Casterline, D., & Croneberg, C. *A dictionary of american sign language on linguistic principles.* Washington, D.C.: Gallaudet College Press, 1965.
60. Streng, A. *Syntax, speech and hearing.* New York: Grune & Stratton, 1972.
61. Wilbur, R., Quigley, S., & Montanelli, D. Conjoined structures in the language of deaf students. *J. Speech Hearing Res.,* 1975, *18,* 319-335.

Chapter 10

1. Abeson, A. Movement and momentum: Government and the education of handicapped children, *Except. Child.,* 1974, *41,* 109-115.
2. Barngrover, E. A study of educators' preferences in special education programs. *Except. Child.,* 1971, *37,* 754-755.
3. Berg, F.S., & Fletcher, S.G. *The hard of hearing child.* New York: Grune & Stratton, 1970.
4. Birch, J.W. *Mainstreaming: Educable mentally retarded children in regular classes.* Minneapolis: University of Minnesota, Leadership Training Institute/Special Education, 1974.
5. Birch, J., & Stevens, G. *Teaching exceptional children in every classroom: Reaching the mentally retarded.* Indianapolis: Bobs Merrill, 1955.
6. Blackman, L.S. Research and the classroom, Mahomet and the mountain revisited. *Except. Child.,* 1972, *38,* 181-191.
7. Bradfield, R.H., Brown, J.C., & Rickert, E.S. The special child in regular classrooms. *Except. Child.,* 1973, *39,* 384-390.
8. Brooks, B.L., & Bransford, L.A. Modification of teachers' attitudes toward exceptional children. *Except. Child.,* 1971, *37,* 259-260.
9. Brown, R. *A first language.* New York: Harper & Row, 1973.
10. Craig, W.N., & Barkuloo, H.W. (Eds.). *Psychologists to deaf children: A developing perspective.* Pittsburgh: University of Pittsburgh, School of Educ., 1968.
11. Craig, W.N., & Salem, J.M. Partial integration of deaf with hearing students: Residential school perspectives. *Am. Ann. Deaf,* 1975, *120,* 28-36.
12. Dailey, R. Dimensions and issues in '74: Tapping the special education grapevine, *Except. Child.,* 1974, *40,* 503-507.
13. Davis, H. (Ed.). The young deaf child; Identification and management. *Acta Otolaryngol.,* 1965, Suppl. 206. (Proceedings)
14. Davis, H., & Silverman, S.R. *Hearing and deafness.* New York: Holt, Rinehart, 1970.

15. Davis, J. Performance of young hearing-impaired children on a test of basic concepts. *J. Speech Hearing Res.* 1974, *17*, 342-350.
16. Elliott, L.L., & Healey, W.C. Selection of achievement test level for hearing-impaired children. *Lang., Speech, Hearing Serv. in Schools*, 1970, *5*, 33-42.
17. Erber, N.P. Evaluation of special hearing aids for deaf children. *J. Speech Hearing Dis.*, 1971, *36*, 527-537.
18. Furth, H.G. *Thinking without language*. New York: Free Press, 1966.
19. Goetzinger, C.P. Effects of small perceptive losses on language and speech discrimination. *Volta Rev.*, 1962, *64*, 408-414.
20. Goldberg, I., & Lippman, L. Plato had a word for it. *Except. Child.*, 1974, *40*, 325-334.
21. Hayes, J. (Ed.). *Cognition and the development of language*. New York: Wiley, 1970b.
22. Healey, W.C. *Standards and guidelines for comprehensive language, speech and hearing programs in the schools*. Washington, D.C.: Am. Speech Hearing Assoc., 1973-1974.
23. Healey, W., & Karp-Nortman, D. *The hearing impaired mentally retarded: Recommendations for action*. Washington, D.C.: Am. Speech Hearing Assoc., 1975
24. Hehir, R.G. Integrating deaf students for career education. *Except. Child.*, 1973, *39*, 611-618.
25. Hudgins, C.V., & Numbers, F.C. An investigation of the intelligibility of the speech of the deaf. *Genet. Psychol. Monogr.*, 1942, *25*, 289-392.
26. Jones, S.A., & Healey, W.C. *Model regulations for school language, speech and hearing programs and services*. Washington, D.C.: Am. Speech Hearing Assoc., 1973.
27. Kennedy, P., & Bruininks, R.H. Social status of hearing impaired children in regular classrooms. *Except. Child.*, 1974, *40*, 336-342.
28. Kodman, F. Educational status of heard of hearing children in the classroom. *J. Speech Hearing Dis.*, 1963, *28*, 297-299.
29. Lenneberg, E.H. Language disorders in children. *Harvard Educ. in Rev.*, 1964, *34*, 152-177.
30. Ling, D. The use of hearing and the teaching of speech. *Teach. Deaf*, 1963, *61*, 59-68.
31. Mann, P.H. (Ed.). *Mainstream special education*. Reston, Va.: Counc. for Except. Child., 1974.
32. Moore, T. (Ed.). *Cognitive development and the acquisition of language*. New York: Academic, 1973.
33. Moores, D. An investigation of the psycholinguistic functioning of deaf adolescents. *Except. Child.*, 1970, *36*, 645-652.
34. Northcott, W.H. Candidate for integration: A hearing impaired child in a nursery school. *Young Child.*, 1970, *25*, 367-381.
35. Northcott, W.H. The integration of young deaf children into ordinary educational programs. *Except. Child.*, 1971, *38*, 29-32.
36. Payne, R., & Murray, C. Principals' attitudes toward integration of the handicapped. *Except. Child.*, 1974, *41*, 123-125.
37. Quay, H.C. Special education: Assumptions, techniques, and evaluative criteria. *Except. Child.*, 1973, *40*, 165-170.
38. Reynolds, I.G. The school adjustment of children with minimal hearing loss. *J. Speech Hearing Dis.*, 1955, *20*, 380-384.
39. Rosenberg, R.A. Misdiagnosis of children with auditory problems. *J. Speech Hearing Dis.*, 1966, *31*, 279-283.
40. Schlesinger, H.S., & Meadow, K.P. Development of maturity in deaf children. *Except. Child.*, 1972, *38*, 461-467.
41. Shotel, J.R., Iano, R.T., & McGettigan, J.F. Teacher attitudes associated with the integration of handicapped children. *Except. Child.*, 1972, *38*, 677-683.
42. Siegel, E. *Special education in the regular classroom*. New York: John Day, 1969.
43. Smith, C. R. Residual hearing and speech production in deaf children. *J. Speech Hearing Res.*, 1975, *18*, 795-811.
44. Weintraub, F. J., Abeson, A.R., & Braddock, D. L. *State law and education of handicapped children: Issues and recommendations*. Arlington, Va.: Counc. for Except. Child., 1971.
45. Young, D., & McConnell, F. Retardation of vocabulary development in hard of hearing children. *Except. Child.*, 1957, *23*, 368-370.

Chapter 11

1. American Organization for the Education of the Hearing Impaired. Characteristics of an

144   Bibliography

adequate auditory/oral program—A guide for parents and educators. *Volta Rev.*, 1975, *77*, 431-435.

2. Boothroyd, A. *Distribution of hearing levels in the student population of Clarke School for the Deaf* (Sensory Aids Res. Proj. #3). Northampton, Ma.: Clarke School for the Deaf, 1970.
3. Calvert, D. R. The deaf child in the seventies, *Volta Rev.*, 1970, *72*, 14-20.
4. Calvert, D. R., & Silverman, S. R. *Speech and deafness*, Washington, D.C.: A.G. Bell Assoc., 1975.
5. Downs, M.P. The deafness management quotient. *H & S Hearing Speech News*, 1974, *42*, 8-9; 26-29.
6. Elliott, L.L., & Armbruster, V.B. Some possible effects of the delay of early treatment of deafness. *J. Speech Hearing Res.*, 1967, *10*, 209-224.
7. Erber, N.P. Speech-envelope cues as an acoustic aid to lipreading for profoundly deaf children. *J. Acous. Soc. Am.*, 1972, *51*, 1224-1227.
8. Erber, N.P. Effects of angle, distance and illumination on visual reception of speech by profoundly deaf children. *J. Speech Hearing Res.*, 1974a, *17*, 99-112.
9. Erber, N.P. Pure-tone thresholds and word-recognition abilities of hearing-impaired children. *J. Speech Hearing Res.*, 1974b, *18*, 194-202.
10. Erber, N.P. Visual perception of speech by deaf children: Recent developments and continuing needs. *J. Speech Hearing Dis.*, 1974c, *39*, 178-185.
11. Goldstein, M.A. *The acoustic method for training of the deaf and hard of hearing child*, St. Louis, Mo.: Laryngoscope Press, 1939.
12. Grammatico, L.F. The development of listening skills. *Volta Rev.*, 1975, *77*, 303-308.
13. Griffith, C. The auditory approach for preschool deaf children. *Volta Rev.*, 1964, *66*, 387-397.
14. Hudgins, C.V. Auditory training: Its possibilities and limitations. *Volta Rev.*, 1954, *56*, 339-349.
15. Joint Committee on Audiol. and Educ. of the Deaf. Guidelines for audiology programs in educational settings for hearing-impaired children. *ASHA*, 1975, *17*, 17-20.
16. Ling. D. Amplification for speech. In D.R. Calvert, & S.R. Silverman, *Speech and deafness*, Washington, D.C.: A.G. Bell Assoc., 1975, pp. 64-88.
17. Moog, J. Language instruction determined by diagnostic observation. *Volta Rev.*, 1975, *77*, 561-570.
18. Pollack, D. Acoupedics: A uni-sensory approach to auditory training. *Volta Rev.*, 1964, *66*, 400-409.
19. Ross, M., & Calvert, D.R. The semantics of deafness. *Volta Rev.*, 1967, *69*, 644-649.
20. Ross, M. Model educational cascade for hearing impaired children, In Nix (Ed.), *Mainstream education of hearing impaired children*. New York: Grune & Stratton, 1976.
21. Stark, R.E. (Ed.). *Sensory capabilities of hearing-impaired children*. Baltimore: University Park Press, 1974.
22. Suchman, R.G. Visual impairment among deaf children. *Arch. Ophthalmol.*, 1967, *77*, 18-21.
23. Whetnall, E., & Fry, D.B. *The deaf child*. London: Wm. Heinemann, 1964.
24. Wilson, G.B., Ross, M., & Calvert, D.R. An experimental study of the semantics of deafness. *Volta Rev.*, 1974, *76*, 408-414.

Chapter 12

1. AB Specialinstrument, POB 270 66 S-102 51, Stockholm, Sweden.
2. Alcorn, S. Development of the Tadoma method for the deaf-blind. *Except. Child.*, 1945, *11*, 117-119.
3. Bishop, M.E., Ringel, R.L., & House, A.S. Orosensory perception in the deaf. *Volta Rev.*, 1972, *74*, 289-298.
4. Burce, R.V. *Bell, Alexander Graham Bell and the conquest of solitude*. Boston: Little, Brown & Col. 1973.
5. Center for Communications Research, 50 West Main Street, Rochester, N.Y. 14614.
6. Cornett, R.O. *Automatic cuer project, cued speech programs*. Washington, D.C.: Gallaudet Coll. (On-going project)
7. Danaher, E.M., Osberger, M.J., & Pickett, J.M. Discrimination of formant frequency transitions in synthetic vowels. *J. Speech Hearing Res.*, 1973, *16*, 439-451.
8. Danaher, E.M., & Pickett, J.M. Some masking effects produced by low-frequency vowel formants in persons with sensorineural hearing loss. *J. Speech Hearing Res.*, 1975, *18*, 261-271.

9. Danhauer, J.L., & Singh, S. A multidimensional scaling analysis of phonemic responses from hard-of-hearing and deaf subjects of three languages. *Lang. Speech*, 1975, *18*, 42-64.

10. Danhauer, J.L., & Singh, S. *Multidimensional speech perception by the hearing impaired*, Baltimore: University Park Press, 1975.

11. Eimas, P., & Morse, P. Individual papers in R.L. Schiefelbusch, & L.L. Lloyd (Eds.), *Language perspectives–Acquisition, retardation and intervention* (Section I. Infant speech perception), Baltimore: University Park Press, 1974.

12. Englemann, S., & Rosov, R. Tactual hearing experiment with deaf and hearing subjects. *Except. Child.*, 1975, *41*, 243-253.

13. Eulenberg, J. Computer Science Dept., Michigan State University, East Lansing, Mi.

14. Fant, G. (Ed.). *Proceedings of a symposium of speech communication ability and profound deafness, Stockholm 1970*. Washington, D.C.: A.G. Bell Assoc., 1972.

15. Fant. G. (Ed.) Speech and hearing defects and aids. In *Proc. Stockholm Speech Communication Seminar 1974*, New York: Wiley & Sons, in press.

16. Fourcin, A., & Abberton, E. *The laryngograph and the voiscope in speech therapy*. London: Phonetics Dept., University Coll., 1974.

17. Foust, K., & Gengel, R. Speech discrimination by sensorineural hearing-impaired persons using a transposer hearing aid. *Scan. Audiol.*, 1973, *2*, 161-170.

18. Gibson, J.J. Observations on active touch. *Psych. Rev.*, 1962, *69*, 477-491.

19. Gibson, J.J. The useful dimensions of sensitivity. *Am. Psychol.*, 1963, *18*, 1-15.

20. Gibson, J.J. *The senses considered as perceptual systems*. Boston: Houghton Mifflin, 1966.

21. Goldberg, A.J. A visual feature indicator for the severely hard of hearing *IEEE Trans. Audio Electroac.* 1972, *20*, 16-22.

22. Goldstein, M. *Personal communication*, Baltimore: Biomedical Engineering Dept., The Johns Hopkins University, 1974.

23. Hill, D.R. An abbreviated guide to planning for speech interaction with machines: The state of the art. *Internat. J. Man-Machine Studies*, 1972, *4*, 373-410.

24. House, A.H., Goldstein, D.P., & Hughes, G.W. Perception of visual transforms of speech stimuli: Learning simple syllables. *Am. Ann. Deaf*, 1968, *113*, 215-221.

25. Johansson, B. The use of the transposer for the management of the deaf child. *Internat. Audiol.*, 1966, *5*, 362-371.

26. Jonathan Allen, Res. Lab. Electronics, Massachusetts Inst. of Tech., Cambridge, Ma.

27. Kirman, J.H. Tactile communication of speech: A review and analysis. *Psychol. Bull.*, 1973, *80*, 54-74.

28. Kirman, J.H. Tactile perception of computer-derived formant patterns from voiced speech. *J. Acoust. Soc. Am.*, 1974, *55*, 163-169.

29. Levitt, H. Speech-processing aids for the deaf: An overview. *IEEE Trans. Audio Electroac.* 1973, *21*, 269-273.

30. Levitt, H., & Nye, R.W. (Eds.) *Sensory training aids for the hearing impaired*. Washington, D.C.: Nat. Acad. Eng. 1971.

31. Liberman, A.M. Perception of the speech code. *Psychol. Rev.*, 1967, *74*, 431-461.

32. Liberman, A.M., Cooper, F.S., Shankweiler, D.P., & Studdert-Kennedy, M. Why are spectrograms hard to read? *Am. Ann. Deaf*, 1968, *113*, 127-133.

33. Liberman, P. On the evolution of language: A unified view. *Cognition*, 1974, *2*, 59-94.

34. Liberman, P. *On the origins of language*, Riverside, N.J.: Macmillan, 1975.

35. Ling, D. Speech discrimination by profoundly deaf children using linear and coding amplifiers. *IEEE Trans. Audio Electroac.*, 1969, *17*, 298-303.

36. Mackenzie, C. *Alexander Graham Bell*. New York: Grossett & Dunlap, 1928.

37. Mazor, H., Simon, H., Schenberg, J., & Levitt, H. *Moderate frequency transposition for the moderately hearing-impaired*. (Report #8, Communic. Sciences Lab., Doctoral prog. in Speech Sciences, Grad. Cr.). To be published in *J. Acous. Soc. Am.*

38. Medical Research Council, Great Britain, *Hearing Aids and Audiometers*. (Special report series 261), London: Her Majesty's Stationery Office, 1947.

39. Miller, J.D., Engebretson, A.M., & DeFilippo, C.L. Preliminary research with a three-channel vibrotactile speech-reception aid for the deaf. In Fant (Ed.), *Proc. Stockholm Speech Communication Seminar 1974*, New York: Wiley & Sons, in press.

40. Newell, (Ed.)., *Speech understanding systems*. New York: American Elsevier, 1973.

41. Nickerson, R., Kalikow, D., & Stevens, K. Computer-aided speech training for the deaf. *J. Speech Hearing Dis.*, 1976, *41*, 120-132.

42. Nickerson, R.A., & Stevens, K.N. Teaching speech to the deaf: Can a computer help? *IEEE Trans. Audio Electroac.*, 1973, *21*, 445-455.

146   Bibliography

43. Nye, P., Haskins Labs., 270 Crown Street, New Haven, Ct.
44. Pascoe, D.P. Frequency responses of hearing aids and their effects on the speech perception of hearing-impaired subjects. *Ann. Otol., Rhinol. & Laryngol.*, 1957, *84*, Suppl. #23.
45. Pickett, J.M. Tactual communication of speech sounds to the deaf: Comparison with lipreading. *J. Speech Hearing Dis.*, 1963, *28*, 315-330.
46. Pickett, J.M. (Ed.). Proceedings of Conference on Speech-Analyzing Aids for the Deaf. *Am. Ann. Deaf*, 1968, *113*, 116-330.
47. Pickett, J.M. Speech science research and speech communication for the deaf In L.E. Connor (Ed.), *Speech for the deaf child: Knowledge and use.* Washington, D.C.: A.G. Bell Assoc., 1971.
48. Pickett, J.M., Gengel, R.W., & Quinn, R. Research with the Upton eyeglass speech-reader. In Fant (Ed.), *Proc. Stockholm Speech Communication Seminar 1974*, New York: Wiley, in press.
49. Pickett, J.M., & Pickett, B.H. Communication of speech sounds by a tactual vocoder. *J. Speech Hearing Res.*, 1963, *6*, 207-222.
50. Piminow, L. Technical and physiological problems in the application of synthetic speech to aural rehabilitation. *Am. Ann. Deaf.* 1968, *113*, 275-282.
51. Potter, R.K., Kopp, G.A., Kopp, H.G. *Visible speech.* New York: Van Nostrand, 1947.
52. Risberg, A. A critical review of work on speech-analyzing hearing aids. *IEEE Trans. Audio Electroac.*, 1969, *17*, 290-297.
53. Saber Foundation, P.O. Box 1055, Cocoa Beach, Fl. 32931.
54. Stark, R.E. (Ed.). Sensory capabilities of hearing-impaired children. Baltimore: University Park Press, 1974.
55. Telesensory Systems, Inc., 2626 Hanover Street, Palo Alto, Ca. 94304.
56. Varispeech Systems, Lexicon, Inc., 60 Turner Street, Waltham, Ma. 02154.
57. Villchur, E. Signal processing to improve speech intelligibility in perceptive deafness. *J. Acoust. Soc. Am.* 1973, *53*, 1646-1657.
58. Walden, B., & Montgomery, A. Dimensions of consonant perception in normal and hearing-impaired listeners. *J. Speech Hearing Res.*, 1975, *18*, 444-455.
59. Walden, B., Prosek, R., & Worthington, D. Auditory and audiovisual feature transmission in hearing-impaired adults. *J. Speech Hearing Res.*, 1975, *18*, 272-280.
60. Willemain, T.R., & Lee, F.F. Tactile pitch displays for the deaf. *IEEE Trans. Audio Electroac.*, 1972, *20*, 9-16.

Chapter 13

1. Anthony, D., (Ed.). *Seeing Essential English Manual.* Anaheim, Ca.: Educ. Serv. Div., Anaheim Union School Dist., 1971.
2. Battison, R. Phonological deletion in American sign language. *Sign Lang. Studies*, 1974, *5*, 1-19.
3. Bellugi, U. Studies in sign language. In T.J. O'Rourke (Ed.), *Psycholinguistics and total communication.* Washington, D.C.: Am. Ann. Deaf, 1972, pp. 68-84.
4. Bender, R.E. *The conquest of deafness.* Cleveland: Western Reserve University Press, 1960.
5. Bornstein, H., (Ed.). *Signed English basic preschool dictionary.* Washington, D.C.: Gallaudet College Press, 1973.
6. Brasel, K., & Quigley, S.P. *The influence of early language and communication environments on the development of language in deaf children.* Urbana: Inst. Res. Except. Child., University of Illinois, 1975.
7. Brill, R. The superior IQs of deaf children of deaf parents. *The California Palms*, 1969, *15*, 1-14.
8. Cicourel, A., & Boese, R. Sign language acquisition and the teaching of deaf children. In D. Hymes, C. Cazden, & V. John (Eds.), *The functions of language: An anthropological and psychological approach.* New York: Teachers Coll. Press, 1972.
9. Denton, D.M. A rationale for total communication. In T.J. O'Rourke (Ed.), *Psycholinguistics and total communication.* Washington, D.C.: Am. Ann Deaf, 1972, pp. 53-61.
10. Fant, L.J., Jr. *Ameslan, an introduction to American sign language.* Silver Spring, Md.: Nat. Assoc. Deaf, 1972.
11. Garretson, M.D. Communicating in international signs. *Gallaudet Today*, 1971, *2*, 8-9.
12. Gustason, G., Pfetzing, D., Zawolkow, E. *Signing exact English: Seeing instead of hearing.* (Rev. ed. 1975). Rossmoor, Ca.: Modern Signs Press, 1972.
13. Hodgson, K.W. *The deaf and their problems.* New York: Philosophical Library, 1954.
14. Holcomb, R.K. Three years of the total approach—1968-1971. *Proceedings of the forty-fifth*

meeting of the Convention of American Instructors of the Deaf. Washington, D.C.: U.S. Govt. Printing Off., 1972, pp. 522-530.
15. Kent, M.S. Total communication at the Maryland School for the Deaf. Deaf Am., 1971, 23, 5-8.
16. Lloyd, G.T. Total communication: Some perspectives and potential problems. Deaf Am., 1975, 27, 13-15.
17. Meadow, K. Early manual communication in relation to the deaf child's intellectual, social, and communicative functioning. Am. Ann. Deaf, 1968, 113, 29-41.
18. Moores, D. Psycholinguistics and deafness. Am. Ann. Deaf, 1970, 115, 37-48.
19. Rogers, E.M. Communication of innovations. New York: Free Press, 1971.
20. Scherer, P. Editorial. Center Dial., 1974, 1, 1-2.
21. Schlesinger, H.S., & Meadow, K.P. Sound and sign: Childhood deafness and mental health. Berkeley, Ca.: University of California Press, 1972.
22. Scouten, E.L. Education and the prelingually deaf child. Deaf Am. 1969, 21, 6-8.
23. Stokoe, W.C., Jr. Sign language studies: An outline of the visual communication systems of the American deaf. Buffalo, N.Y.: University of Buffalo Press, 1960.
24. Stokoe, W.C., Jr. The study of sign language. Washington, D.C.: Cr. for Applied Ling., 1970.
25. Stokoe, W.C., Jr. CAL conference on sign languages. Ling. Reporter, 1970, 12, 5-8.
26. Stuckless, E.R., & Birch, J.W. The influence of early manual communication on the linguistic development of deaf children. Am. Ann. Deaf, 1966, 111, 452-460.
27. Switzer, M.E. On the frontier of silence: The moral obligation to communicate. Washington, D.C.: Soc. Rehab. Serv., HEW, 1968.
28. Vernon, M., & Koh, S.D. Effects of early manual communication on achievement of deaf children. Am. Ann Deaf, 1970, 115, 527-536.
29. Vernon, M., & Koh, S.D. Effects of oral preschool compared to early manual communication in education and communication in deaf children. Am. Ann. Deaf, 1971, 116, 569-574.
30. Vernon, M., & Makowsky, B. Deafness and minority group dynamics. Deaf Am., 1969, 21, 3-6.
31. Wampler, D. Linguistics of Visual English. Santa Rosa, Ca.: Early Childhood Educ. Dept., Aurally Handicapped Prog., Santa Rosa City Schools, 1971.

Chapter 11

1. Bellugi, U., & Klima, E.S. The roots of language in the sign talk of the deaf. Psychol. Today. June, 1972, 61-76.
2. Bornstein, H. Signed English: A manual approach to English language development. J. Speech Hearing Dis. 1974, 39, 330-343.
3. Brasel, K.E., & Quigley, S.P. The influence of early language and communication environments on the development of language in deaf children. Champaign: University of Illinois, Inst. Res. Except. Child., 1975.
4. Corson, H. Comparing deaf children of oral deaf parents and deaf parents using manual communication with deaf children of hearing parents on academic, social, and communicative functioning. Doctoral dissertation, Cincinnati: University of Cincinnati, 1973.
5. Crandall, K.E. English functor morphemes used in Signed English by deaf children and their parents. Proceedings of the Annual Meeting of Am. Speech Hearing Assoc., Washington, D.C., 1975.
6. Ellenberger, R.L., Moores, D.F., & Hoffmeister, R.J. Early stages in the acquisition of negation by a deaf child of deaf parents. (Res. Rep. #94). Minneapolis: University of Minnesota, Res., Develpm., & Demon. Ctr. in Educ. Handicapped Child., 1975.
7. Gates, R. The reception of verbal information by deaf students through a television medium—A comparison of speechreading, manual communication, and reading. In Proceedings, Conv. of Am. Instr. of the Deaf. Little Rock, Ar., Washington, D.C.: Am. Ann. Deaf, 1971, pp. 513-522.
8. Hammermeister, F.K. Reading achievement in deaf adults. Am. Ann. Deaf, 1971, 116, 25-28.
9. Hoemann, H. The development of communication skills in deaf and hearing children. Child Develpm. 1972, 43, 990-1003.
10. Hoemann, H., & Tweney, R. Is the sign language of the deaf an adequate communication channel? In Proceedings, Conv. of American Psychol. Assoc., Vol. II. Montreal, Canada, 1973, 801.

11. Moores, D.F. *Recent research on manual communication*. Occasional Paper no. 7. Minneapolis: University of Minnesota. Res., Develpm., & Training Cr. in Educ. of Handicapped, 1971.
12. Nix, G. Total communication: A review of the studies offered in its support. *Volta Rev.*, 1975, 77, 470-494.
13. Norwood, M. *Relative effectiveness of interpreted and captioned news among deaf adults.* Paper presented at NTID Mini-Convention, Nat. Tech. Inst. for Deaf. Rochester, N.Y., 1976.
14. Panko, J. *The learning effects of visual mediated verbal presentation formats on deaf postsecondary students.* Doctoral dissertation, Pittsburgh: University of Pittsburgh, 1975.
15. Propp, G. *An experimental study on the encoding of verbal information for visual transmission to the hearing impaired learner.* Doctoral dissertation, Lincoln: University of Nebraska, 1972.
16. Quigley, S.P. Language acquisition. *Volta Rev.*, 1966, 68, 68-83.
17. Quigley, S.P., Wilbur, R.B., Power, D.J., Montanelli, D.S., & Steinkamp, M.W. *Syntactic structures in the language of deaf children.* Champaign: University of Illinois, Inst. Child. Beh. & Develpm., 1976.
18. Stuckless, E.R. *An interpretive review of research on manual communication in the education of deaf children: Language development and information transmission.* London: Royal Nat. Inst. for Deaf, in press.
19. Weiss, K.L., Goodwin, M.W., & Moores, D.F. *Characteristics of young deaf children and early intervention programs* (Res. Rep. #91). Minneapolis: University of Minnesota, Res. Develpm., & Training Cr. in Educ. of Handicapped, 1975.
20. White, A., & Stevenson, V. The effects of total communication, manual communication, oral communication and reading on the learning of factual information in residential school deaf children. *Am. Ann. Deaf*, 1975, 120, 48-57.

Chapter 15

1. Cornett, O.R. *Cued speech parent training and follow-up program* (Contract # OEC-8009137-4348(019) and (615)). Washington, D.C.: Gallaudet Coll. Off. of Educ., 1972 (Final Report).
2. Englemann, S., & Rosov, R. Tactual hearing experiment with deaf and hearing subjects. *Except. Child.*, 1975, 41, 243-253.
3. Gault, R.H., & Crane, G.W. Tactual patterns from certain vowel qualities instrumentally communicated from a speaker to a subject's fingers. *J. Gen. Psychol.* 1928, 1, 353-359.
4. Geldard, F.A. *Vision, audition, and beyond in contributions to sensory physiology*, (Vol. 4). New York: Academic Press, 1970.
5. Helmholtz, H.L.F. *Popular scientific lectures.* New York: Longmans, Green, 1881, p. 116. (Pg. refer. to reprint, Dover, N.Y., 1962)
6. Helmholtz, H.L.F. *On the sensations of tone.* New York: Longmans, Green, 1885, p. 173. (Pg. refer. to reprint, Dover, N.Y., 1954)
7. Saunders, F.A., Hill, W.A., & Simpson, C.A. *Hearing substitution: A wearable electrotactile vocoder for the deaf.* (USPHS 5 501 RR 05566-08 and NINCDS, NS 09714). Washington, D.C.: Public House Service.
8. Sherrick, C.E. Sensory Processes. In J.A. Swets, & L.L. Elliott (Eds.), *Psychology and the handicapped child*, Washington, D.C.: U.S. Govt. Printing Off., 1974, p. 34.
9. Stepp, R.E. *A feasibility study to investigate the instrumentation, establishment, and operation of a learning laboratory for hard of hearing children* (OE3-16-0044 NDEA Title VII-B). Washington, D.C.: Off. of Educ., 1965. (Final Report)
10. Upton, H. Wearable eyeglass speech reading aid (Proc. Conf. on Speech-Analyzing Aids for the Deaf). *Am. Ann. Deaf*, 1968, 113, 222-229.
11. Withrow, F.B. Field testing of the Withrow Noun Vocabulary Films. *AOEHI Bull.*, Winter, 1969, p. 3-8.

Chapter 16

1. Schein, J.D., & Delk, M.T. *The deaf population of the United States.* Silver Spring, Md.: Nat. Assoc. Deaf, 1974.

Chapter 17   8816069

1. Fournier, J.E. Hearing aid evaluation by pure tone automatic audiometry. *Audecibel*, 1968, 17, 99-108.
2. Pascoe, D.P. Frequency responses of hearing aids and their effects on the speech perception of hearing impaired subjects. *Ann. Otol., Rhinol., Laryngol.* 1975, 84, suppl. 23.